Couple Work, Work with Couples

Couple Work, Work with Couples provides a new exploration of psychoanalysis with couples. Éric Smadja takes two key approaches, first providing a metapsychological exploration of couple work – at intrapsychic-individual, intersubjective and group levels – and investigating love, being in love and the principal structural phases and psychic organisers of couples, then exploring the work of the choice of conjugal object and its historicity. He also introduces and develops useful notions such as intertransferential neurosis at work at the intersubjective level. Smadja continues by rethinking psycho-analytic work with couples, with reference to the work of leading French psychoanalysts, group analysts and couple analysts. The book highlights specific features of working with couples, such as the creation of a specific analytic situation – "the therapeutic group" – and then considers the benefits and expected effects of this kind of work.

With clinical material from the author's work throughout, *Couple Work, Work with Couples* will appeal to psychoanalysts and psychoanalytically informed clinicians working with couples.

Éric Smadja is a psychiatrist and psychoanalyst (working with adults and couples) based in Paris, France. He is a member of the Société psychana-lytique de Paris and of the International Psychoanalytical Association. He is also the founder of a specific training in psychoanalysis with couples and an anthropologist. In 2007, he was awarded the IPA Prize for "Exceptional Contribution made to Psychoanalytical Research".

The International Psychoanalytical Association Current Challenges in Psychoanalysis Series

Series Editor: Silvia Flechner

IPA Publications Committee

Natacha Delgado, Nergis Güleç, Thomas Marcacci, Carlos Moguillansky, Rafael Mondrzak, Angela M. Vuotto, Gabriela Legorreta (consultant)

Recent titles in the Series include

Psychoanalysis and Severe Disorders in Young Children
Clinical and Community Work with Autism Spectrum Disorder and Child Mental Health
Nahir Bonifacino

Couple Work, Work with Couples
Éric Smadja

Couple Work, Work with Couples

Éric Smadja

Routledge
Taylor & Francis Group

LONDON AND NEW YORK

Designed cover image: Getty | IssaraJarukitjaroon

First published 2025
by Routledge
4 Park Square, Milton Park, Abingdon, Oxon OX14 4RN

and by Routledge
605 Third Avenue, New York, NY 10158

Routledge is an imprint of the Taylor & Francis Group, an informa business

© 2025 Éric Smadja

British Library Cataloguing-in-Publication Data
A catalogue record for this book is available from the British Library

ISBN: 978-1-041-06370-4 (hbk)
ISBN: 978-1-041-06369-8 (pbk)
ISBN: 978-1-003-63509-3 (ebk)

DOI: 10.4324/9781003635093

Typeset in Palatino
by Taylor & Francis Books

Contents

Series editor's foreword

The International Psychoanalytic Association Publications Committee is honoured to present a new book from the Current Challenges in Psychoanalysis series.

This series delves into the evolving landscape of psychoanalytic practice, addressing contemporary issues such as trauma, cultural diversity, technology's influence and shifts in psychoanalytical dynamics. Each volume offers concise, interdisciplinary insights from leading experts, bridging classical psychoanalytic theory with modern challenges. Designed for clinicians and researchers, this series is a vital resource for those seeking to navigate and innovate within today's complex therapeutic environment.

The IPA Publications Committee is pleased to publish Dr Éric Smadja's book *Couple Work, Work with Couples*. In this new book, Dr Smadja revisits couples from the perspective of their psychic reality and envisages, on the one hand, the modalities of a metapsychological exploration based on the reflections of authors not known as couple specialists but inspiring and stimulating in this new research. On the other hand, he rethinks psychoanalytic work with couples, relying on the writings of individual psychoanalysts, group analysts and analysts of couples.

Dr Éric Smadja is a psychiatrist and psychoanalyst who works with adults and couples in Paris. He is a member of the Société psychanalytique de Paris and the International Psychoanalytical Association. He is also an anthropologist. His work is psychoanalytic and interdisciplinary. This book explores the theoretical point of view of couple work and the clinical psychoanalytic work with couples. It was first published in French by Éditions InPress, France.

The book addresses the couple's central time, psychic organisers and choice of the conjugal object. It then explores the conjugal psychic reality at its three levels – group, intersubjective, and individual-intrapsychic – through "couple work".

The author immerses us in the couple's conflict, love, and being in love, the principal structural phases and psychic organisers of couples, and the work of the choice of conjugal object and its historicity. The author also discusses the technical and tactical aspects of the analyst's work and specific aspects of his or her own psychic work in session with a couple.

The Publications Committee is interested in sharing this new book with the psychoanalytic community and other related disciplines to expand their knowledge and allow acquaintance with the author.

Silvia Flechner

Series Editor

Chair, IPA Publications Committee

Introduction

More than ten years have now passed since, in *Le couple et son histoire*,[1] I began an exploration of the couple using a pluri- and interdisciplinary approach integrating history, anthropology, sociology and psycho-analysis. There, I told several stories: the sociocultural story of the couple that began with the institution of marriage; the story of the couple's construction as an object of knowledge and psychoanalytic treatment, the foundations of which were laid by Sigmund Freud, then Melanie Klein, D. W. Winnicott and W. Bion; the story of the couple's conjugal life cycle, from the time the two partners meet until their ageing together; and lastly the story of suffering couples who go to consult a couple therapist and undertake joint psychoanalytic work.

It was a matter of the initial *organising* and *shaping the contours* of an investigation, endeavouring then to develop a general, unified and intelligible, though inevitably heterogeneous, portrayal of the couple.

In addition, I laid down some foundations there and introduced notions and concepts, such as:

- The couple's multidimensional, sexual-bodily, sociocultural and psychic reality, the last of these being organised in accordance with three structuro-functional levels: groupal, intersubjective and intrapsychic-individual.
- The couple's essentially ambivalent, conflictual and critical nature.
- The notion of intertransferential neurosis that every couple partially constitutes on the intersubjective level.
- The couple's structural external conflictualities of a historical and socio-cultural nature and internal conflictualities of an intrapsychic-individual as well as intersubjective nature.
- Couple work.
- The concept of conjugal culture and of conjugal identity.
- The foundations of a specific technique for working with couples.

Then, in 2013, in *Couples en psychanalyse*,[2] I invited some fellow couple therapists to present, through an account of an experience of therapy,

DOI: 10.4324/9781003635093-1

either a conjugal issue inherent to the natural life cycle of every couple, such as the erotic life, the desire for a child and the critical stage of the birth of a child, or a frequently encountered painful situation such as conjugal violence and extraconjugality.

These two works thus form a diptych.

Ten years have already elapsed since then, and time passes so fast …! Those years were marked, notably, by a number of publications developing certain aspects of the couple and by travelling to give lectures and training seminars – in the course of which I presented my ideas about couples and psychoanalytic work with couples, and had the opportunity to enter into contact with a very stimulating variety of colleagues and publics. In addition I, of course, pursued my activity as a couple psychoanalyst and reader of works, which inevitably and necessarily nourished and enriched my thoughts about this reality, which I was increasingly viewing as being much more complex.

However, the anthropologist that I am also strongly felt that age-old desire to work on other research objects, notably on Freudian conceptions of society and culture (*Freud et la culture*, 2013),[3] then on a *fragment* of the history of ideas in the human and social sciences regarding the paths to the discovery of symbolism and symbolisation, both individual and collective – a revolutionary discovery made by those founding fathers of the human and social sciences, Freud, Durkheim and Mauss. This was the subject for my book *On Symbolism and Symbolisation: The Work of Freud, Durkheim and Mauss* (2018).[4]

Since then, my investigative drive, still just as lively, *impelled* me to revisit couples, this time exclusively from the perspective of their psychic reality, and to envisage on the one hand the modalities of a metapsychological exploration based on the reflections of authors not known as couple specialists, but nevertheless intensely inspiring and stimulating in this new research pursuit. I will name, in particular, S. Freud, M. Klein, D. W. Winnicott, W. Bion, D. Anzieu, G. Bayle, M. Bouvet, C. David, J. L. Donnet, M. Fain, A. Green, B. Grunberger, R. Kaës, E. Kestemberg, S. Lebovici, P. Luquet, P. Marty, M. De M'Uzan, C. Parat, P. C. Racamier, B. Rosenberg, R. Roussillon and J. Schaeffer.

And, on the other hand, I felt impelled to rethink psychoanalytic work with couples, relying also on the writings of individual psychoanalysts (J. L. Donnet, P. Denis, A. Green and M. Neyraut), group analysts (D. Anzieu and R. Kaës), and couples analysts (J. G. Lemaire).

Indeed, all these authors helped me revisit the three "structuro-functional" levels I had already partially identified, differentiated and explored.

Benefitting from such diverse, rich and fruitful conceptual elaborations, I was ultimately better able to find my way within this universe, which is so complex, as much in terms of the plurality and heterogeneity of its materials, as by its topics. These are composed of multiple spaces, strata and networks of relations of interdependence. The dynamic of this couple psychic reality is plural and multilocal, animated by forces, conflictualities. Its psychic economy is pervaded by currents of drive investments so different in nature.

As for my work with couples, I have been able to think and theorise about my method, the characteristics of the analytic situation with couples – producing in particular a *therapeutic group*, the role of which will be fundamental – its framework, the processual dynamic, as well as the particularities of the transfero-countertransferential dynamic, certain characteristics of the analyst at work, and certain technical aspects of my work, whether tactical and interpretative, always in reference to individual work and to work with groups.

I am therefore proposing two major sides of a diptych: The first will involve the metapsychological exploration of couple work on the three structuro-functional levels: intrapsychic-individual, intersubjective and groupal (Part I, Chapters 2, 3 and 4).

This exploration will be preceded by an introduction recalling what is essential about the concept of couple work, and by Part I, Chapter 1 devoted to love, being in love and to the principal structural phases and psychic organisers of couples, followed by the work of the choice of conjugal object and its historicity.

This exploration will close with a final chapter, Part I, Chapter 5, devoted to the role played by couple work in the temporality of the couple. Indeed, we suggest some metapsychological reflections, then we discuss its critical dimension, a few evolving perspectives, the conditions of its durability and the elaboration of an investigation into the question of the separation of the two partners and the correlative breaking up of the couple.

Allow me to add that I will not be discussing the complex and heterogeneous universe of homosexual couples, male or female, particularly because I think that their couple work does not differ greatly from that of heterosexual couples. The economic, dynamic and topical aspects, whether intrapsychic-individual, intersubjective or groupal, display great similarities. Moreover, living together as a couple poses the same fundamental sets of problems for homosexuals and heterosexuals. One of the major differences concerns the type of choice of object, heterosexual or homosexual, with its own historicity.

Furthermore, we must definitely differentiate couples in love or conjugal couples from those who have become parental couples. However, my exploration of couple work at the three structuro-functional levels will not distinguish between them specifically. Rather, I will be able to reflect on the economic and dynamic relationships between the conjugal-love and parental dimension of every couple within the framework of couple work.

The second side will deal with the work with couples that is conditioned and sustained by this metapsychological approach. It begins with methodological and epistemological introductory considerations and then presents a first clinical chapter, Part II, Chapter 1, devoted to the diversity of the circumstances of the consultation of suffering couples. While Part II, Chapter 2 looks at making contact with the analyst, the preliminary interviews or the "encounter", then the criteria for evaluating and making a decision about working with couples. Finally, the last chapter (Part II, Chapter 3) develops the technical aspects, both tactical and strategic, of the analyst's work, as well as certain aspects of his or her own psychic work in session with a couple. The characteristics of the interpretative activity will be illustrated by a fairly stimulating clinical situation, which will be followed by the expected effects and benefits of work with couples.

It is now time to discover this exploration.

Notes

1 É. Smadja, *Le couple et son histoire* (Presses universitaires de France, 2011, in French); as *The Couple: A Pluridisciplinary Story* (Routledge, 2016, in English).
2 É. Smadja (ed.), *Couples en psychanalyse* (Presses universitaires de France, 2013).
3 É. Smadja, *Freud et la culture* (Presses universitaires de France, 2013, in French); as *Freud and culture* (Karnac and IPA, 2015, in English).
4 É. Smadja, *On Symbolism and Symbolisation: The Work of Freud, Durkheim and Mauss* (Routledge, 2018).

Part I
Couple work

Introduction to Part I

Recalling the concept of couple work

The construction of a couple and its *living* durability proceeds from work that is not only of a psychic order, but also of a sexual-bodily and sociocultural order. It is a matter of couple work, a concept I introduced in 2011 in *Le couple et son histoire*.[1] Let us recall what it is essential about this concept with regard to its multidimensionality, its failures and its functions.

This interdisciplinary concept of couple work helps us to interpret conjugal facts pertaining to each one of the three realities – sexual-bodily, psychic and sociocultural – endowed with their own temporality. It also helps us to understand their necessary connections as well as their insufficiencies.

This couple work is realised conjointly by the partners' Ego, in the service of couple's interests which is invested for a more or less important part. This work mobilises the three levels of conscious, pre-conscious and unconscious and involves economic, dynamic and topical aspects. It is therefore accomplished within the three realities of the couple described above, the temporality of each of these realities conditioning that of the corresponding work.

This couple work must be able to conflictualise and realise economic, dynamic and flexible connections among the three realities, thus ensuring tolerable, durable and satisfactory conjugal functioning, both for the couple and for its members.

Nevertheless, it is inconceivable apart from its structural (therefore, ongoing) antagonism with each partner's individual work ("work of the individual") realised at the service of each one. So, over the course of time, how will each one's Ego distribute its investments between individual work and couple work? In other words, what portions will it be able to devote to itself and to the couple? Moreover, inevitable differences will spring up between the two partners with respect to this antagonism regarding the preferential investment of one conjugal reality or another, differences which will or will not be compensated for by the partner's work. These differences will probably vary during the course of the conjugal cycle, but they will also appear to be fixed in place, something that runs the risk of causing conjugal difficulties.

DOI: 10.4324/9781003635093-3

In the sociocultural reality

The conjugal couple must necessarily also constitute a "work couple", which will supply it with the material means of its social existence, positioning it in the vast, complex, stratified, differentiated social structure.

Thus, couple work will involve work in the home, conjugal socialisation work, parental work (when the conjugal couple becomes a parental couple), among other forms of work, to fit into the more general framework of work for the development of a conjugal culture and identity, made possible by the preliminary work accomplished within the psychic reality.

Referring back to the ideas of W. R. Bion[2] and D. Anzieu[3] about groups, this "work couple" or "technical pole" (in Anzieu) therefore corresponds to one of two levels of conjugal functioning. The other level would be the fantasised couple in interrelationship with it, which will nourish it with fantasies, drive investments, and also limit it by means of anxieties and defensive measures. It therefore represents a form of voluntary, conscious cooperation between the two partners in the accomplishment of different common tasks relating to the couple's material and social existence. For Bion and Anzieu, it would involve the Ego's characteristics, here the "conjugal Ego" governed by the reality principle and animated by the logic of the functioning of the secondary psychic processes. This cooperation is obviously not exclusively rational, "secondarised", but also permeated, even disturbed, by a paralysing or stimulating, conscious and unconscious, fantasised and emotional flow.

Within the sociocultural reality

Couple work consists in: investing and maintaining narcissistic, erotic, tender and aggressive investments of the other person's body; constructing representations of separate sexual bodies, and a "fantasy of psycho-bodily pairing"; identifying with the other person, mobilising one's own psychic bisexuality for that; communicating narcissistic, erotic, tender, aggressive messages in diverse ways (for example, verbally and non-verbally, behaviourally, mimetic-gesturally), all of them finding expression, in particular, in a capacity to be concerned about the other person's body, to be seduced by his or her body, to seduce it with one's own body, also to reject it as if an alarm bell is going off.

A question arises about the fate of "psychosomatic organisations" in the course of conjugal life. Would they be better protected from disorganising trauma when couple work is satisfactory, meaning when it can act as a protective shield.

On the contrary, would the bodily repercussions of couple work be potentially pernicious, because traumatogenic, therefore, disorganising – thus expressing the failure of this work? Reflection upon a "couple psychosomatics" needs to be undertaken, inquiring in particular into the role of the couple and couple work, through its diverse modes of participation in the psychosomatic economy of the partners. Inversely, one might enquire into the repercussions of somatic disorganisation experienced by one of the members on the three levels of conjugal reality, something needing to be expanded upon at a later stage of research.

What about the couple's sexuality?

Diversified in its repertory of practices, the couple's sexuality procures aggressive, erotic (pregenital and genital), narcissistic satisfactions. In heterosexual couples, the two libidinal currents – heterosexual and homosexual – will be able to be satisfied, directly in the first case, and through fantasising by identification with the partner in the second case. Its investment will vary as a function of the conjugal culture, the stages of the conjugal cycle, the evolution of each of the partners and of the economy of its investments, and the evolution of certain aspects of their intersubjective relationship, in particular. It will be able to achieve a certain balance with each one's autoerotic sexuality.

Psychoanalytic discourse discusses the realisation of a state of narcissistic completeness (B. Grunberger),[4] reassurance about its narcissistic integrity (A. Green),[5] the acquisition of a feeling of psychic security, experiencing oneself as "good" (M. Klein),[6] and also the realisation of the fantasy of an "imaginary common body", the fantasy of bisexuality denying the difference between the sexes, castration and alterity. However, it also emphasises the necessary underlying psychic work, individual work (J. Schaeffer's "female work", for example)[7] combining with that of the partner mobilising the difference between the sexes, each one's bisexuality, multiple identifications, coping with pregenital and genital anxieties, the specific conflicts between the erotic dimension – with the retentive nature of desire, and that of instinctual discharge – but also between sexuality and the narcissistic desire not to differentiate, and finally that between sexuality and self-preservation.

In sexual-bodily temporality, there is an inevitable discrepancy between the psychic and sociocultural temporalities. This discrepancy is a source of conflict and anxiety, above all, as the partners age. Couple work endeavours to resolve them through adjustments and better connections between the three realities making up the couple.

Within psychic reality

Let us recall the three levels: group, intersubjective, and intrapsychic-individual.

The groupal level

A *conjugal group* exists when a shared, common psychic construction occurs between the partners, a "conjugal psyche" that will function as such from then on and will, in particular, produce "conjugal compromise formations", themselves common and shared. It therefore results from work to synergise and conflictualise the parts of every individual psyche mobilised to construct this conjugal group. It is also made up with the combination of offensive, defensive and structuring unconscious alliances (R. Kaës, 2009).[8]

The convergence of the two partners' fantasies and their unifying elaboration would lead to compromise formations, such as ideologies, mythologies, utopias (Anzieu, 1975)[9] that will orient and determine the general representations of conjugal life, the daily activities, plans, just as they will have an impact on the different types of work realised and, finally, on the elaboration of a conjugal culture and identity.

This *conjugal group* is also endowed with a "fantasised, common and shared living body", the place where its psyche dwells. The couple is, indeed, fantasised by both its members not only as a "womb-like living body", but also invested as a living, growing being that has functional and psychic vital needs to satisfy and will inevitably go through mutative and maturing critical periods.

The intersubjective level

The *intersubjective space* animated by a multifaceted conflictuality connects each partner's object-relations, realises an interplay of identifications and projections contributing to the creation of unconscious alliances and establishes a reciprocal relationship between the two partners' OEdipus and sibling complexes, which contributes to partially constituting an intertransferential neurosis.

The intrapsychic-individual level

This space is also animated by multiple anxiety-generating conflicts and correlative defensive measures that each partner will have to attempt to resolve in order to accept to enter into the conjugal relationship and co-create the conjugal group. These occur between Ego and love-object, Ego and couple-object, between love-object and couple-object, identity and otherness, but also between each one's shareable and unshareable objects.

Couple work's impact upon both partners and its failures

One understands each partner's conjugal life as the expression of the necessary dynamic interconnection between couple work and individual work, each having its respective share combining with the effects of the partner's couple work. Would it rather be beneficial for certain people and detrimental for others? The answer is also tied to the existence of possible failures of couple work. What would they then be?

There are diverse manners of conceiving of them.

Quantitatively speaking, one may point to insufficient Ego work on the part of both parties, or on the part of one of the two, which are not compensated for by the other's work. They may concern one or several realities, the result being experienced as unsatisfactory by one or both partners, potentially conflictual with hostile projective movements, which will lead to conjugal suffering.

What do I mean by excessive couple work? We can understand this as a predominant investment in this work on the part of the Ego of one or both of the partners to the detriment of individual work, something which will have harmful individual repercussions at a later point with consequences for the couple. This can, furthermore, be a matter of the overinvestment of one or several realities to the detriment of others, making this economically costly with potentially disorganising effects owing to later impairment of the work.

Qualitatively speaking, one may point to aspects that are systematic, fixed in place (and therefore not very flexible or easy to mobilise) and not creative enough, modalities of accomplishing this work independently of the realities (sexual-bodily, psychic or sociocultural).

I will also look at work to establish connections between these three realities, work that may be insufficient or excessive, as well as work providing consistency and harmonisation among the temporalities that relate to each.

This couple work and its failures inevitably raise questions about the notions of normality and pathology in the couples' lives together, about its functions, its evolution over the course of individual and conjugal time.

Some functions corresponding to each of the three levels of reality

Psychic functions

Besides its functions of providing the members of a couple with very regressive, direct narcissistic satisfactions – symbiotic and fusional aspirations – and also with fantasised satisfactions through male and female identifications made possible by the mobilisation of each partner's bisexuality, couple work also responds to protective defensive needs vis-à-vis internal dangers (pregenital drives, homosexuality, destructive drives, multiple pregenital and oedipal fantasies and anxieties) and external dangers (projected conflictual or persecutory objects) that are satisfied by making unconscious defensive alliances (denegative pacts). Moreover, in subjects with a fragile social, psychic organisation, it would make it possible to provide a "framework", a structuring function, suggesting to me the function of the "auxiliary Ego" of a mother for her infant.

However, one of the major functions of couple work is also to foster a certain durability of conjugal life, outside of any form of suffering (psychic, social and sexual-bodily).

Finally, I want to mention the couple's function of repairing early narcissistic wounds.

Sexual-bodily functions

Apart from the protection of the psychosomatic organisation and the durable twofold investment – narcissistic and erotic – of his or her own body and that of the other person reciprocally, there are the direct erotic, tender, aggressive, pregenital and genital, heterosexual satisfactions as well as the homosexual satisfactions, fantasised through identification with the partner. The strengthening of conjugal identity and that of the sexual component of the identity of each of the partners is also to be associated with this.

Sociocultural functions

As I have already explained, the couple and its work must ensure its material and social existence, produce the means to achieve that, and satisfy its needs in this conjugal domain. It must create a conjugal culture conferring a singular identity upon the couple. When the couple becomes a parental couple, it must engage in parental and family work – for example, childrearing.

Finally, couple work must conflictualise these three levels by establishing dynamic liaisons and economically balanced investments of a libidinal and self-preserving nature.

Having come to the end of this review, we must now take a look at the preliminary and founding experiences and phases, those of love and of being in love, then the phases and psychic organisers of the construction of every couple, integrating of course historicity and the diverse modalities of the work of the choice of conjugal object.

Notes

1   É. Smadja, *Le couple et son histoire* (Presses universitaires de France, 2011, in French); as *The Couple: A Pluridisciplinary Story* (Routledge, 2016, in English).
2   W. R. Bion, *Experiences in Groups and Other Papers* (Tavistock Publications, 1961).
3   D. Anzieu, *The Group and the Unconscious* (Routledge, 1999; first published 1975).
4   B. Grunberger, *Le narcissisme* (Payot & Rivages, 1993; first published 1971).
5   A. Green, *The Chains of Eros: The Sexual in Psychoanalysis* (Karnac, 2008). Translation of *Les chaînes d'Eros, l'actualité du sexuel* (Odile Jacob, 1997).
6   M. Klein, "Love, guilt and reparation", in Melanie Klein and Joan Riviere (eds), *Love, Hate and Reparation* (W. W. Norton, 1964; first published 1937).
7   J. Schaeffer, *Le refus du féminin* (Presses universitaires de France, 1997).
8   R. Kaës, *Les alliances inconscientes* (Dunod, 2009).
9   D. Anzieu, *The Group and the Unconscious* (Routledge, 1999; first published 1975).

1 Love, being in love, structural phases and psychic organisers of couples, and the work of the choice of conjugal object and its historicity

Love and being in love

Catherine Parat (1967)[1] reminds us that oedipal love corresponds to the first model of love that did not attain drive realisation, but only satisfaction of a tender and sublimated kind. However, the inevitable and necessary renunciation of the first object of love constitutes an objectal and narcissistic failure for the child, which will leave its mark on adult love.

An essential characteristic of this adult love relation consists, she considers, "in synthesising a still (that is to say, since the time of the oedipal emotion) known portion of old emotions and a radically new portion of emotions, adult love partly establishing itself on the former oedipal desire".[2]

For his part, C. David (1971)[3] invites us to consider love as a *mixed entity* within which he discerns a share of repetition (repetition compulsion) and a share of innovation, of narcissism and of objectality, of expansive tendency to synthesis and of internal antagonism, the idea of a specific interhuman bond and of transferential manifestation, of restructuring regressive movement and of defence.

In fact, this shared state leads to the formation of a new bond and to a metamorphosis of the individual psyches, "but also, owing to the crossed projections and identifications, to the constitution of a relational dyad. Love will be both an outcome, but also the pursuit of a great organising and evolving movement".[4]

Existing and developing in parallel in each of the lovers is, according to David, a nostalgia for the primordial mother-child dyad combining with the oedipal wound, with unconscious guilt and ambivalence. "Primary" love, with its pregenital oral, anal and phallic components and its oedipal aspects, underlies our various loves when we reach maturity.

David defines being in love as

> a dynamic constellation of conscious and unconscious desires, feelings, fantasies and affects which for a time modifies the three dimensions – dynamic, economic and topical – of the subject's psychic organisation and finds expression in an irresistible disposition to constitute the chosen

DOI: 10.4324/9781003635093-4

object as source and center of all satisfaction, of all happiness, mobilising the essential of its drive economy.[5]

This also involves reviving a set of affects and of *transferred* old desires as well as beginning a new life.

This intertransferential and transferential dimension between the two persons in love is to be emphasised, and later on we will explore its importance and its implications for the structuring of every couple.

Finally, with reference on one hand to the scars left by the oedipal conflicts and on the other hand to the interminable pubertal waiting, the "surprise of love" and being in love bring delayed compensation as well as unconsciously constituting revenge on the parental couple, formerly frustrating just by its very existence and by the reality of complicity among adults, as well as reparation, which can be considered a triumph and comes late to compensate for the ineluctable feeling of failure due to effective powerlessness.

"The narcissistic wound, as well as the trauma of eviction, both finally find their true remedy".[6]

However, in the lovers' unconscious, these joys of being in love, with their unconscious meanings of late triumph, revenge and reparation, also represent a differed realisation of formerly impossible transgressions. Whence an unconscious feeling of guilt always seems present when in love.

Structural phases and unconscious psychic organisers of the construction of the couple

What are the unconscious psychic motivations impelling us to seek being in love and to form a couple?

How does one choose one's conjugal and love partner?

Why choose this or that partner rather than another at such a time in one's life?

I consider that:

- The first phase of nostalgia for the maternal primary object relation, therefore that of the primordial mother-child dyad (a space of mutual primary identification and a source of narcissistic completeness and integrity for the child), is connected with the censorship of the woman as lover, bearer of fantasies of seduction and of the primal scene.
- The second phase is that of the OEdipus complex and its correlate, the oedipal organisation of the genital stage, inscribed in the diphasism of sexuality, with its pubertal and childhood phases separated by the period of latency.
- Finally there is the sibling complex, nested in the OEdipus complex.

These constitute the structural phases and the fundamental unconscious psychic organisers which contribute to the construction of every couple.

Let us acquaint ourselves with these structural phases.

Relation to the maternal primary object

This nostalgic pursuit of the relation to the maternal primary object would correspond to the desire to satisfy our originary fantasy of returning to the foetal state, to the mother's womb, therefore, to the foeto-maternal fusion, but also to the "mother-infant unit" described by D. W. Winnicott.[7]

Let us not forget that Freud spoke of the mother not only as a person who feeds and cares for her child, but also as arousing in it a good number of unpleasant or pleasant bodily sensations. The mother is then the first seducer of the child, of *her* child, something that will leave indelible mnesic traces in the child.

He expressed this very clearly in his *Outline of Psychoanalysis* (1940) in this way:

> A child's first erotic object is the mother's breast that nourishes it; love has its origin in attachment to the satisfied need for nourishment [...]. By her care of the child's body she becomes its first seducer. In these two relations lies the root of a mother's importance, unique, without parallel, laid down unalterably for a whole lifetime, as the first and strongest love object and as the prototype of all later love relations – for both sexes.[8]

From B. Grunberger's (1971) perspective,[9] this search for "narcissistic union" with the partner would aim at "reestablishing the narcissistic integrity" lost too early by each one of us and would produce a state of "narcissistic completeness" expressed through the phallic image in the partners' unconscious.

P.-C. Racamier (1995)[10] studied the mutual mother-child "narcissistic seduction" following the prenatal bodily unity or foeto-maternal fusion to constitute a unity together in which each party recognises itself.

This mother-child narcissistic relationship, aiming to constitute an omnipotent unity, naturally enters into an antagonistic relationship with the "forces of growth" that induce differentiation, separation and autonomy. According to Racamier, it is a matter of the "antoedipal" conflict, that of the origins, thus setting the forces of narcissistic seduction against those of growth, something observable in any couple.

There in fact exists both a seduction of a narcissistic kind – setting into motion the primary narcissism and the processes of primary identification of the mother and the child, aiming to reconstitute the omnipotent foeto-maternal unity – and an objectal seduction of an erotic kind, each of them being recognised and appreciated in its otherness and its singularity, as well as an individual need for differentiation and separation.

This "antoedipal" conflict would then be reactivated in every couple.

In a couple, we are looking for, and we sometimes find, at certain particular times, these diverse aspects of this primary and primordial relationship as well as some other ones to be discovered now.

Let us recall with A. Green (1990)[11] that *the mother must play the role of auxiliary Ego, drive container and mirror for the child.* And let us also look at *the role of the maternal protective shield and the censorship of the woman as lover* with M. Fain (1971).[12] "For a mother having a normally developed maternal instinct, the baby has an Ego, that of its mother, a capacity to love, that of its mother".[13]

Indeed, when the mother is present, she invests her baby's id that, owing to this, becomes (only partly) her Ego. This investment of the newborn by its mother is accompanied by a narcissistic withdrawal going to the point of "maternalising the milieu". A primary identification is then formed by the mother and the child. The drive source proper to the child is thus situated inside the "mothering system" and within the primary identification. The mother plays a role of protective shield for her baby and would also be responsible for the organisation of primary repression.

However, in spite of this maternal investment, a part of her libido remains distinctly erotic, that is to say a woman subsists somewhere who creates a forbidden zone within this mothering milieu, the couple's bedroom. So, temporarily disinvesting her child as soon as desire transforms her into a woman, she breaks off the primary identification and in so doing frees the drive potentialities of her child's id.

Thus, *the censorship of the mother as lover* will immediately act on these potentialities, which may interfere with the paternal desire, so as to give it free rein, and the maternal disinvestment will drive her child to shape representations which will resonate with the originary fantasies (seduction and primordial scene).

"The mother and the woman will always remain irreconcilable enemies".[14]

From that time on, the child becomes a nuisance whose id is to be silenced, neutralised. To rid herself of it, she is going to have to rock her child to sleep. Censorship and representations will result in keeping the child asleep, resuming the role of protective shield – sleep that will distance it from paternal desire.

The censorship of the woman as lover above all seeks to protect this paternal desire situated outside the psychic apparatus, but exercising this censorship inscribes the place of this desire within the child's id, in fact confirms a situation inscribed within the existence of the originary fantasy.

Thus, each partner will be able, will have to be able, to play, alternatively or simultaneously, with the other partner, the maternal roles of auxiliary Ego, of drive container, of protective shield and of mirror, making it possible to "psychise" the traumatic experience of each of their love lives, but also to help the other person reinforce his or her counterinvestments, whence is found the defensive function sought after and accomplished by each member of the couple.

As for *the censorship of the woman as lover*, conceptualised by Fain, it seems to me to contain one of the primary psychic determinants of the constitution of the couple. Indeed, when the mother disinvests her child in order to invest her narcissism and the father's desire, thus transforming herself into a woman as lover, she introduces her child to an early oedipal triangulation and to a future primal scene, something that would play a role in the underlying causes of the desire for a future couple through early hysterical identification with the desire of the mother who has once again become the father's lover.

Let us now look at this role of primary mirror described by Winnicott, which was then taken up again by Green and developed in a remarkable way by R. Roussillon (2008)[15] with the introduction of his model of a "mirror primary homosexuality" (homosensuality).

If, in the beginning, this model concerns the organisation of the mother-baby primary relation, it nonetheless presupposes that the "basis" of this first relation would remain present and more or less active all throughout life, whence its presumed underlying presence, active and sought after in every conjugal relationship, which is the source of all its interest.

What is it specifically a matter of and in what respect would it play a role in the conjugal dynamic?

According to Roussillon, the first forms of satisfaction and of organisation of the first bond, the "basis" of the experience of satisfaction, presupposes the constructing and the encountering of an object that is a "double" of oneself, formed after the model of the child's unified narcissism.

A "double" is both the same and other, which rules out indifferentiation and psychic confusion. This "double" makes itself, and is made to be, similar in the encounter and the conditions of the latter.

For a certain quality of the "mirrored homosexual" pleasure to exist, the other person must be encountered as being someone similar who accepts *sharing the same existential states, the same psychic states*. This is the role of the mother, but also that which is sought for in the conjugal and love partner.

Roussillon considers that the process by which each of the two partners is constituted as a mirror and double of the other one must establish itself on two intertwined levels. The first level is that of an "aesthetic" sharing and of a sharing of bodily sensations. It is here that it can be said to be "homosensual". This level forms the basis upon which the second level is going to be established, that of affective harmonising and of emotional sharing. This process would thus condition the "mirrored homosexual" pleasure and its psychic components.

The OEdipus complex

According to Parat (1967), the OEdipus complex represents, "the psychic conflict which creates a really new libidinal structuration. It constitutes the hub of human evolution, institutes a new mode of being, of feeling, of thinking, of communicating with other people".[16]

Oedipal triangulation constitutes an attempt to group the tender affects and the erotic desires onto the heterosexual object and the hateful affects onto the object of the same sex. However, the homosexual object will at the same time remain only a rival, an object of love and a model.

Oedipal triangulation leads above all to the love investment of an object of the opposite sex, that is to say for the boy and for the girl, "to the recognition and to the valorisation in love of the difference between the sexes".[17]

However, this drive movement leads to failure owing to the renunciation of the object of desire for reasons that are as superegoic (fear of castration for the boy, fear of the loss of the mother's love for the girl) as they are due to "inevolution" – owing to each one's need to preserve the object of identification of the same sex – as well as those connected with the *inadequacy of the object*, being based on the gap between the psychic and physical maturation between the subject and the object, something constituting the narcissistic traumatism of the oedipal failure.

This is why drive satisfaction, the realisation of the child's oedipal desire, can only be something virtual, at the acme of its first oedipal impulse. The child is then "locked into virtuality".[18]

As a consequence, the oedipal conflict involves both a "constant and inevitable major objectal frustration combined with narcissistic failure" that will leave "a trace which rightly marks our humanity, and whose indelible mark can be found as long as life lasts".[19]

As Fain (1967)[20] has suggested, this oedipal failure is at play in libidinal evolution like a point of fixation.

David (1967)[21] confers *mutative and structuring value upon the totality of the diphasism* governing the establishing of human sexuality, something I also recognise and accept as unconscious psychic organiser of every couple.

Latency

From the structural point of view, it occurs as a period of increasing autonomy, of firming up and of economic preponderance of the Ego, and also as that which sees the Superego constituted as a specific and independent agency.

One then sees the child fighting against the world of his or her drives and in particular fighting against his or her sex drive, using a great part of the rest of his or her available forces for the implementation of the Ego's synthetic function, still not very operative at the beginning of latency.

A decrease in the sexual activities, along with a more or less forceful desexualisation of objectal relations and of affects, as well as an unbinding of narcissistic and objectal libidinal currents then occurs.

Erotic desire – which persists as an unconscious current – transforms into tender love. There exist the beginnings of sublimation and of new reaction-formations. After going through the period of latency, at the time of pubertal blossoming, modified sexual drives are going to reappear through the work of the period of latency, but also a revitalisation of the oedipal conflicts and affects, as well as a limiting of the consequences of the oedipal failure.

Adolescence

E. Kestemberg (1999)[22] considers that while everything is prepared during childhood, even in very early childhood, it all plays out in adolescence, the "afterwardness" or "*après coup*" of which is characteristic, something which is of particular interest to me with regard to the historicity of the choice of conjugal and love-object. This period during which the adult's destiny is played out occurs at a time when each individual's body is definitively sexualised.

Adolescence seems to Kestemberg to play a mutative and organising role from childhood to adulthood and represents considerable psychic work of elaboration of the field of very diverse forces, at the end of which the adolescent become adult will have had to:

- integrate a new image of a sexualised body, therefore renounce possessing the two sexes;
- secure new sources of regulating his or her inner tensions and pleasures which take into account his or her access to the possibility of sexual relations, in connection with his or her infantile sexuality, such as it has been able to organise itself around his or her erogenous zones and the organising inner objects of his or her infantile neurosis;
- secure for him- or herself a regulation of self-esteem that is more independent of his or her immediate entourage, in the constitution of which the metamorphoses of the connections with the first objects, post-oedipal superegoic interiorisations, are integrated as the ideals of the milieu in which he or she is going to evolve.[23]

It is the process of becoming autonomous of one's parents and, therefore, of identification, which is at stake.

However, Kestemberg also emphasises that adolescence has "traumatic" potentiality because of the access to the possibility of sexual genital activity and of the demands of psychic work represented by the impulses of the sexual drive and the transformations of the body that these demands imply.

What has then become of the oedipal object of desire during the genital impulses of adolescence?

Parat (1967) states that, beginning with puberty, the object invested is no longer the oedipal object, because one of the movements of adolescence precisely consists of the detachment from the parental objects necessary for "the young man or girl to reach adult status, that is to say, affective freedom, with the opportunity to invest a love-object other than the oedi-pal parent or a substitute".[24]

Consequently, these different rearrangements, which concern both the sexual drives and the love-object, will lead to the possibility of establish-ing a love relationship, part of which will not be built on the former oedipal desire.

In the classic cases, all these affects are going to find themselves directed towards the same heterosexual object. Genital satisfaction, when it will be able to develop itself, is going to find itself accompanied and doubled by homosexual and pregenital satisfactions, the love-object finding itself invested in different ways. However, the *oedipal fixation* ensures the con-tinued existence of the oedipal conflict and the failure of the first genital oedipal impulse, often while denying the conflict. If a fixation exists, the object invested in fact remains the parental oedipal object, or a direct (parental or sibling) substitute of the latter.

The oedipal organisation of the genital stage

This oedipal organisation of the genital stage (Parat, 1967)[25] corresponds to a mode of libidinal structuration stemming from the oedipal triangulation, which realises the genital stage and maintains the distribution of the affects in two sectors, one being occupied by the heterosexual object, the other being fulfilled by "the others", outside the couple.

It thus includes a double relationship in a three-way system:

- A *heterosexual relationship* which groups and synthesises a genital cur-rent, a tender sentimental current, and a pregenital current, in favour of a real object towards which these currents are drawn and which is neither the oedipal parent, nor a substitute for this parent.
- A homosexual relationship is established with the outside world, with "reality" constituted by all the others.

This double relationship of course presupposes the existence of corre-sponding internal objects, and the relationship with real objects always including movements of projection and movements of introjection.[26]

I will examine more fully these two types of *interactive relationships* during our exploration of the intersubjective level, then its temporal dynamic in Part I, Chapter 5 devoted to the temporality of the couple.

The couple-object and the OEdipus complex

According to Roussillon (2008),[27] the couple is an "object", the construc-tion and investment of which also have a history in the adult and child libidinal economy.

When at the beginning of the child's oedipal conflict, they are confronted with the narcissistic impasses of the organisation of their auto-erotic drive life, the oedipal child is going to transfer the realisation of their ideal onto the representation of the couple of their reunited parents, the pivotal moment of which would be to be situated in the organisation of the fantasy of the primal scene.

For the oedipal child, the couple then becomes this "all in one" ideal object in which the two sexes can be united, where discharge and pleasure of discharge are combined with the bond and pleasure of the binding.

Considered separately, the father as much as the mother will have demonstrated their shortcomings, however joined together in a couple they form an omnipotent entity.

This couple-object invented by the child is an object that is at once narcissistic, omnipotent and objectalising, allowing every child to come out of their autoerotic position in order to go towards the other person and to form with this other person an omnipotent couple in the likeness of the invented couple-object.

Confronted with the reality of their parental couple, the oedipal child can then begin to differentiate the internal couple-object they created from the perception of the actual couple, thus leading to the elaboration of an idealised internal and actual parental couple double, something enabling them to acquire a certain amount of independence vis-à-vis the perceived couple of their parents and, according to Roussillon, a certain "dissolution" of the OEdipus complex would be conceivable, consisting of this distribution over two different scenes of the relationship to the actual couple and the relationship to the internal representation of the couple-object, as such transferable on to different objects.

It is easily imaginable that the invention of this omnipotent couple-object will also help the oedipal child to attenuate the narcissistic traumatism of the oedipal failure, as well as contributing through transference to the construction of its couple in adulthood.

I thus detect a historicity within the psychic construction of the couple and of the choice of conjugal object, marked, as I had already indicated, by different structural phases and unconscious psychic organisers. Let us now take them up more specifically.

An initial *organising phase* corresponds to the *foeto-maternal fusion* followed by the system made up of the mother-child couple and of the censorship of the woman as lover, which mobilises the narcissistic and primary identifications. The originary fantasies are already at work, among them the intra-uterine fantasy, then the seduction and primal scene fantasies with the censorship of the woman as lover.

This is followed by an initial *phase of latency* of a narcissistic and auto-erotic kind, dominated by organ pleasure and pregenital drives, up until the *OEdipus complex. The OEdipus complex, initial genital impulse* – with its double, narcissistic and objectal failure and the construction of an omnipotent "couple-object" – represents the *second organising phase*, accompanied by fantasies of seduction, of primal scene and of castration.

It will produce, "if everything goes well", the *oedipal organisation of the genital stage*, which involves a double relation, heterosexual (with the chosen object, which is no longer the oedipal object) and homosexual (with the external world), this whole then forming a three-way system stemming from the oedipal triangulation.

The period of latency, strictly speaking, that of pubertal waiting, constitutes a *second phase of latency*, which is followed by the *third organising phase*, that of *pubertal and adolescent blossoming*, with its sexual bodily transformations and its psychic reorganisations finally making it possible for the adolescent psychically and physically to realise his oedipal and primary desires.

However, a *fourth organising phase* would be constituted by a final determinant transition, that of *reaching adulthood*, which presupposes the overcoming of the critical trials of adolescence, as well as of the possibilities of definitive choice of love-object and of construction of an adult couple, different from the adolescent couple.

Let us finally take a look at the last organiser of the couple.

The sibling complex

In this regard, why consider the sibling complex to be another unconscious psychic organiser of couple?

As R. Kaës (2008)[28] points out, the sibling complex confronts us with this *other narcissistic double and perhaps bisexualised fellow human being*, who occupies the fantasised place of a brother or sister in our inner world. If the sibling complex is a psychic organiser of sibling bonds, within any group as well as within any couple, so also sibling intertransferential movements composed of love, of rivalry, of jealousy, of hatred and of envy in particular are going to occur between the partners, reviving modes of infantile sibling object relationships, whence the role of the sibling complex as specific and complementary organiser of the couple.

Moreover, the notion of primary homosexuality elaborated by Kestemberg (1984)[29] and that of "mirrored homosexuality" (homosensuality) suggested and developed by Roussillon (2008),[30] refer us also to certain aspects of the sibling complex in this structuring relationship, to the narcissistic double and to the sharing of the same sensations, emotions, thoughts and fantasies. Moreover, the couple is this space where this experience with the fellow human being, this narcissistic and bisexualised double, can be relived, or lived for the first time.

"So it is that one enters into the couple as much by the OEdipus complex as by the sibling complex", to paraphrase Kaës.[31]

What does Kaës tell us specifically about the sibling complex?

Kaës (2008) considers that the sibling complex's specificity comes from its organisation and from its function. Its structure is organised in conjunction with attraction, desire, love and curiosity, and also with rivalry, jealousy, envy, hatred and the rejection that a subject feels vis-à-vis this other fellow human being who, in his or her inner world, occupies the fantasised place of a brother or a sister.

The sibling complex takes on meaning in the process of the constitution of the Ego, of narcissism and identifications with the other fellow human being, just as its values and functions take on meaning in every subject's psychosexual organisation. "The sibling complex is nested in the OEdipus complex, but for fundamental reasons they do not merge with each other".[32]

Kaës distinguishes two main forms of the sibling complex, an archaic form and an oedipalised form:

- The fixations on the imagos and figures of the narcissistic double, of homosexuality and of sibling or "adelphic" bisexuality refer to the archaic sibling complex.
- The archaic forms of the sibling complex are born in the psychic space, the place of which is the mother's fantasised body filled with brothers and sisters, as partial objects and not differentiated subjects.

Among the principal figures of the double that the clinic of sibling complex gives us, the most frequent one is *the specular narcissistic double*, brother or sister, the perfect form of oneself that mirrors the brother for the sister and the sister for the brother chosen.

Kaës considers psychic bisexuality to be a complication of the narcissistic double. As identification, it implies the establishment of otherness. However, an area of overlap exists between the narcissistic double and the bisexual double. The sister and the wife are two figures of feminine doubles for a man, the narcissistic double and the double that should fulfil his bisexual fantasy.

This sibling complex evolves from the archaic towards the oedipal, the symbolical, when the brothers and sisters are symbolically separated and detached from their mother's body and consequently recognised as distinct and total objects.

The recognition of the otherness and of the vital coordination of the parental and of the sibling refers *to the oedipalised sibling complex*.

The oedipal accomplishment of the sibling complex requires a double movement of identifications: the identification with the fellow person of the same generation, sharing the same origin, i.e., the narcissistic component of the identification; and the identification with the parent of the same sex, which at the same time preserves the bisexual component of the identifications with the father and with the mother.

I will not go further into sibling love and incestuous fantasy nor into the affects of hatred, envy and jealousy, which are components active in the sibling complex. Moreover, while from the psychic point of view sibling bonds are organised by the sibling complex, Kaës considers that the latter has an existence and a consistency independently of sibling bonds.

Finally, the sibling complex is modified upon the death of the parents. It is reactivated with the birth of one's own children and with all the major transformations of life that put us back in touch with childhood.

We must now take a more comprehensive look at the historicity and the diverse modalities of the choice of conjugal and love-object, which results from genuine psychic work.

Historicity and work of the choice of conjugal object

Before we start, let us recall the mutative and structuring value connected with the totality of the diphasism governing the establishment of human sexuality. This evolution in two phases in fact conditions the obligation of renouncing the object of oedipal love, which is definitely an object lost forever though nonetheless sought after.

The different rearrangements of the work of the period of latency and of adolescence, which concern both the sexual drives and the love-object, will especially involve *work of detaching, of disinvesting the real parental objects*, opening up the possibility of investing a future love-object other than the oedipal parent or a direct (parental or sibling) substitute; therefore, of being able to establish a love relationship, a part of which will not be built on the former oedipal desire.

According to David (1971), it will have to display affinities with regard to what is old and malleability with regard to what is new. "Finding a love object is re-finding it, as Freud said, but it is also discovering it and practically inventing it",[33] as David emphasises, which suggests the (re) created-(re)found object of Winnicott.

This is obviously so, but Green (1967) gives us some details regarding this, which prove to be both illuminating and quite necessary. He maintains that it is the repressed threat of castration

> that will be the cause of the orientation of the attachment to *another object*, responsible, as we know, for finding certain of the traits there which have most decisively marked the oedipal object. It matters little that these traits can be the very ones which will jeopardise the new union by awakening the threat of castration is of little importance. What is essential is that the *return* of the first attachment finds a way to realisation.[34]

This return is quite obviously that of the repressed representation of the oedipal object.

In fact, though responsible for the decline of the OEdipus complex, the threat of castration also proves to be its protector, to the extent that the need to abandon the forbidden object and to put sexuality on hold during latency would permit

> the later rebirth of an attachment not exhausted in its investment, in search of a new object which will have the double advantage of being different from the first, therefore other, and yet united to it through a bond of partial identity.[35]

Thus, the future love-object of adolescence, and of adulthood above all, will on the one hand be different from the oedipal object, necessarily other, and on the other hand nevertheless include bonds of partial identity.

This love-object will then take on the structure of a compromise formation, which is a matter of genuine psychic work having begun even before the period of latency.

What we ultimately discover with these authors, and with Green in particular, is principally *the reality of psychic work determining the future choice of love-object of adulthood.* As we have already envisaged it, that of adolescence occurs during a critical period that will lead to a kind of defensive choice, narcissistic in this case, involving a significant portion of homosexual investments.

From this perspective, the work of J.-G. Lemaire, pursuing those of Freud and M. Klein, has established in a determinant manner, notably in his *Le couple, sa vie, sa mort* (1979), the different modalities of the choice of conjugal object by introducing certain completely new ones into it and by insisting on its dual polarity, both as a source of multiple sorts of satisfactions (narcissistic, erotic, tender and aggressive) and as serving to reinforce the defensive organisation of the Ego of each one of the partners.

The different choices of object according to J.-G. Lemaire

In relationships of the conjugal kind, that is to say based on the dual polarity of satisfaction and defence, Lemaire considers that

> the object selected must therefore correspond both to positive characteristics, like every object in every love relationship, but it must in addition present determinant complementary characteristics, those enabling the subject to maintain its unity, the coherence and the defense of its Ego, in short, its stability and its security in face of inner threats connected with the persistence of repressed, persisting, drive currents. Thus, what the subject selects among the characteristics of his or her future partner, besides common opportunities for satisfaction, is his or her capacity for participating in his or her defensive organisation, principally in the areas in which he or she falls short. This is undoubtedly the most general law determining the particularities of the choice of principal partner in the conjugal relationship.[36]

These diverse types of choice take up again and develop the three unconscious psychic organisers that I have identified and discussed, but also
present others, of a defensive kind. In addition, these choices of object are
part of a systemic conjugal dynamic that develops the Kleinian intuition of
a correspondence between the two partners' unconsciousness.

Choice referred back to the parental imagos (that is to say, oedipal choice)

One easily finds in this kind of choice the trace of the duly repressed
incestuous desires for each parent. The OEdipus, in its negative and positive forms, leaves its mark there.

- Either in the choice of object, by substitution referred directly back to
  one of the parental figures.
- Or in a defensive, indirect form, where the Subject seeks to use a
  future partner to better protect him- or herself against excessively
  intense oedipal desires repressed in the unconscious, but not yet
  overcome.

So, we will distinguish:

- The choice of the partner in direct reference, whether positive, or
  negative, back to the parental image of the parent of the opposite sex.
- And the choice of the partner in reference to the image of the parent of
  the same sex mobilising the partner's psychic bisexuality.

We will also discuss *the choice in reference to negative and positive images of
the parental couple.*

Choice of narcissistic object integrating one of the destinies of the homosexual libido

According to Freud, one can choose in the partner what one oneself is,
what one oneself was, what one oneself would like to be, according to
one's Ego Ideal and the person who is or was a part of oneself.

This narcissistic choice is in fact favoured by the unconscious homosexual components and facilitates mutual co-identification. This modality
of choice is frequent in adolescents in particular.

Let us now look at some types of defensive choices.

Defensive choice of object and pregenital drives

The love-object is therefore used as a means of protection against the diverse
expressions of partial (sadistic, masochistic, voyeuristic or exhibitionist)

drives, not, or poorly, integrated into the instinctual whole and having to be kept repressed and counterinvested.

Choice of defect

It is a matter of a completely new modality of object choice that had not previously been identified.

Some narcissistic benefits can also be drawn from the choice of negative characteristics in the partner. In these cases, it is the latent defect of the object that is chosen along the same lines that the subjects themselves fear is defective about themselves: depressive tendencies, impulsiveness, social, intellectual or affective capabilities. It would be a matter of carrying over to the partner the defect that one fears in oneself.

Thus, a sense of self-worth emerges thanks to this more defective partner.

Choice of partner as protection against the risk of an intense love and to avoid being swallowed up or devoured by a love-object that is too absorbing

A poorer relationship, or a more ambivalent one mixed with a little hatred, is less feared and can sometimes be considered to be protective. So it is that some subjects can be led to choose their partner principally in order to avoid being swallowed up or devoured.

For certain people, this perception of danger is accompanied by symptoms of either a psychic nature (for example, anxiety or aggressiveness) or a somatic nature (impotency, frigidity, headaches, etc.). In others, this perception is expressed in quasi-preventive behaviour such as keeping the chosen object at a distance, maintaining a large number of activities or emotional and affective involvements outside the main partner or preventive multiplication of extraconjugal partners.

This defensive strategy impels the subject to choose, unknowingly, an object displaying analogous perceptions. This is why the introduction of a third separating and protecting factor into their relational space is observable in these couples.

Choice of partner as external support of the persecutory, bad interiorised objects

The issues involved in the relationship with a partner invested as a bad object are always complex and unstable, since the partner cannot only be invested in that way, but always in association with other more positive modes of investment.

In general, this partner is initially an object of desire invested as good in an ambivalent way, which, however, is inversed later on. His or her narcissistic investment must last for at least a longer amount of time than his or her characteristic of being a bad object, a source of frustration and persecution.

Certain subjects habitually suffering from significant relational difficulties behave as if they need a partner to hate, in the absence of which they would succumb to greater difficulties, and notably into a persecution delirium or a persecutory experience accompanied by corresponding behavioural troubles. Indeed, it is good to recognise the presence of such issues to one degree or another within most couples, since one day they will tend to manifest themselves in a more or less veiled manner.

I consider these issues to arise habitually in many couples in a minor way when it is a matter of using the partner and the couple as a space for rubbish, a place and system of healthy discharge of a persecutory experience, of a great amount psychic excitation connected with the multiple wounds and frustrations of daily life not directly relating to the partner.

The example of Judith and Albert

Judith and Albert, both in their 30s, met at their first motorcycle class. Mother of two girls by two different men, working in the teaching profession, Judith appears to be intellectual, cultivated and exhibit emotional mastery.

Albert, the father of a teenage girl, is a "sales person". He appears to be infantile, funny, not very cultivated and particularly impulsive.

In this couple, one finds a combination of several types of the choices already mentioned. The reference to the parental couple, positive for Albert, and negative for Judith; the choice of a weakness sought for on a certain level in Albert by Judith, that of affective and emotional fragility, particularly finding expression in impulsiveness and violent outbursts that leave an impression upon her and fascinate her. She would have a tendency to induce them, unconsciously of course. She would in fact take advantage of these violent outbursts, which are directed against her as well, to indulge her fantasies by identifying with him, all the while confirming for herself that she is better than him, meaning stronger than him, and more serious, by criticising him and condemning him for that transgression. One discovers that Judith displays the same dispositions as Albert, but they are repressed and counterinvested. She was never able to explode in the way she fantasised. But in his angry outbursts, Albert identifies with his violent father, whom he feared. He also behaves like an unruly, irascible child, with Judith representing a superego mother figure making him feel guilty. Actually, after his impulsive outbursts, Albert feels unhappy, ashamed and guilty, like a bad son and a bad, disappointing companion, the whole thing probably satisfying significant masochistic dispositions in him. While Judith is attracted by this fragility on the part of Albert, for him, she represents an ideal figure, through her emotional mastery, her intelligence, her cultivation and her facility in speaking. But she talks too much and floods him with her speeches "which bore him to death". The protection against the risk of intense, invasive love finds expression in him through a regular need to distance himself from her through his work, which leads him to absent himself from the couple for days at a time. In her case, this distance finds expression in her need to place between the two of them the fathers of her two daughters, with whom she maintains special friendships, causing Albert to feel jealous. Finally, let me underline a distinctly marked homosexual component in their couple, finding expression in masculinity on Judith's part, which attracts Albert, as well as a certain femininity on his part, which seduces her particularly. They are like two buddies who have fun together.

Having identified these structural phases and unconscious psychic organisers of the couple, as well as the historicity and the diverse modalities of the work of choosing a conjugal and love-object, I propose to examine the couple work operative within each of the three structuro-functional levels of conjugal psychic reality.

Notes

1 C. Parat, "L'organisation œdipienne du stade genital", *Revue française de psychanalyse*, 31, 5–6 (1967), pp. 802–803.
2 C. Parat, "L'organisation œdipienne du stade genital", *Revue française de psychanalyse*, 31, 5–6 (1967), pp. 802–803.
3 C. David, *L'état amoureux* (Payot, 1971), p. 211.
4 C. David, *L'état amoureux* (Payot, 1971), p. 211.
5 C. David, *L'état amoureux* (Payot, 1971), p. 45.
6 C. David, *L'état amoureux* (Payot, 1971), p. 187.
7 D. W. Winnicott, *The Maturational Processes and the Facilitating Environment* (Hogarth Press, 1965).
8 S. Freud, *Abrégé de psychanalyse* (1940), OCF.P, XX, 1937–1939 (Presses universitaires de France, 2010), p. 283. From Freud's *An Outline of Psychoanalyis* as translated in D. W. Winnicott, *Playing and Reality* (Routledge, 2005; first published 1971).
9 B. Grunberger, *Narcissism, Psychoanalytic Essays* (International Universities Press, 1979). Translation of Béla Grunberger, *Le narcissisme* (Payot, 1971).
10 P.-C. Racamier, *L'inceste et l'incestuel* (Les éditions du Collège, 1995).
11 A. Green, *La folie privée* (Gallimard, 1990).
12 M. Fain, "Prélude à la vie fantasmatique", *Revue française de psychanalyse*, 35, 2–3 (1971).
13 M. Fain, "Prélude à la vie fantasmatique", *Revue française de psychanalyse*, 35, 2–3 (1971), p. 320.
14 M. Fain, "Prélude à la vie fantasmatique", *Revue française de psychanalyse*, 35, 2–3 (1971), p. 320.
15 R. Roussillon, *Le jeu et l'entre-je(u)* (Presses universitaires de France, 2008).
16 C. Parat, "L'organisation œdipienne du stade genital", *Revue française de psychanalyse*, 31, 5–6 (1967), p. 795.
17 C. Parat, "L'organisation œdipienne du stade genital", *Revue française de psychanalyse*, 31, 5–6 (1967), pp. 796–797.

18 C. Parat, "L'organisation œdipienne du stade genital", *Revue française de psychanalyse*, 31, 5–6 (1967), p. 797.
19 C. Parat, "L'organisation œdipienne du stade genital", *Revue française de psychanalyse*, 31, 5–6 (1967), p. 795.
20 C. Parat, "L'organisation œdipienne du stade genital", *Revue française de psychanalyse*, 31, 5–6 (1967). Response to C. Parat's report.
21 C. Parat, "L'organisation œdipienne du stade genital", *Revue française de psychanalyse*, 31, 5–6 (1967), "De la valeur mutative des remaniements post-oedipiens". Response to C. Parat's report.
22 E. Kestemberg, *L'adolescence à vif* (Presses universitaires de France, 1999).
23 E. Kestemberg, *L'adolescence à vif* (Presses universitaires de France, 1999), pp. 170–171.
24 C. Parat, "L'organisation œdipienne du stade genital", *Revue française de psychanalyse*, 31, 5–6 (1967), p. 764.
25 C. Parat, "L'organisation œdipienne du stade genital", *Revue française de psychanalyse*, 31, 5–6 (1967).
26 C. Parat, "L'organisation œdipienne du stade genital", *Revue française de psychanalyse*, 31, 5–6 (1967), p. 769.
27 R. Roussillon, *Le jeu et l'entre-je(u)* (Presses universitaires de France, 2008).
28 R. Kaës, *Le complexe fraternel* (Dunod, 2008).
29 E. Kestemberg, "'Astrid' ou homosexualité, identité, adolescence", in *L'adolescence à vif* (Presses universitaires de France, 1999; first published 1984).
30 R. Roussillon, *Le jeu et l'entre-je(u)* (Presses universitaires de France, 2008).
31 R. Kaës, *Le complexe fraternel* (Dunod, 2008).
32 R. Kaës. *Le complexe fraternel* (Dunod, 2008), p. 217.
33 C. David, *L'état amoureux* (Payot, 1971), p. 64.
34 A. Green, "Les fondements différenciateurs des images parentales, Intervention sur le rapport de C. Parat", *Revue française de psychanalyse*, 31, 5–6 (1967), 896–897.
35 A. Green, "Les fondements différenciateurs des images parentales, Intervention sur le rapport de C. Parat", *Revue française de psychanalyse*, 31, 5–6 (1967), 897.
36 J.-G. Lemaire, *Le couple, sa vie, sa mort* (Payot, 1979), p. 66.

2   Couple work on the intrapsychic-individual level

On this level, I look at the couple work operative in the inevitably conflictual relationships of each partner's Ego with respect to its two new objects, love-object and couple-object (external and internal, perceived and represented), as well as between those two objects. It will be more clearly understood through the organisation of the Ego, its drives and its internal objects, in accordance with a metapsychological exploration dealing with the economic, dynamic and topic aspects.

However, let us remain aware that it is the totality of each one's psychic apparatus (first and second topic) that is quite obviously engaged in this couple work. In addition, let us keep in mind that this couple work, accomplished by each partner's Ego to serve the couple's interests, always maintains an antagonistic relationship with the individual's work or individual work realised to serve each one's interests. This is what we will discover with the work-object.

Before starting, I will review some fundamental facts about the Ego and its objectal environment in order to contextualise the presence within it of its two new objects which the couple work will especially have to help to integrate while limiting the defensive reactions of individual work in particular.

The Ego (topic, dynamic and economy)

Let us recall that the Ego is an essential agency of conflict (A. Green, 1973),[1] a conciliator and organiser of discharges and adjustments of the relationship. It is also an organisation directly tied to objectal relationships and its functions can be modified by those objectal relationships (P. Luquet, 2003).[2]

Its topical situation splits it into two irreconcilable parts. Indeed, at the intersection of external and internal reality, or through its dual orientation, it is torn between the Ego-pleasure and the Ego-reality. In addition, the Ego is caught between two fronts: that of its drives, always supposed to be contained, and that of the object, too often indeterminate, considered as the more dangerous, because one must take into account of one's drives, which transpire in relation with it (Green, 1973).[3]

DOI: 10.4324/9781003635093-5

The functioning of the Ego enables one to distinguish diverse levels (Green, 1993):[4]

1   A mode of action vis-à-vis drives.
2   A functioning in relationship to its internal organisation.
3   Outwardly oriented activity.

Consequently, the Ego of each partner engaged in a conjugal relationship will have to act on its own drives as well as establish and organise its (external and internal) objectal relations and, moreover, manage its internal functioning.

Among its principal functions, let us mention: the perception and recognition of external reality; the preservation of self-preservation; narcissistic investment conferring the Ego's narcissistic organisation; desexualisation; identification; the defence mechanisms whose roles are multiple; the linking of free energy and the mastering of affects (Green, 1973).[5] Finally, the synthetic function of the Ego creates bonds among all its different currents. These are energising, dynamic syntheses of self-maintenance. A basic energising level is thus ensured so as to feed and maintain the Ego's dynamics. The contributions come from the id and are only maintained in the Ego through fantasising. Outside of it, there are only diverse discharges (G. Bayle, 2012).[6]

In contrast to the anarchic and disorderly regime of investments of the id, the Ego possesses a network of stable investments at a constant level. It is an organisation functioning with the energy converted by relative desexualisation. It serves to constitute the specific aspect of the investments of the Ego: self-preservation, guaranteeing its limits and cohesion, solidifying its consistency. This energy will also serve couple work's different operations.

The Ego and its objects

The metapsychological couple drive/object

"No one is without object. No one is what it is without object', declared Green (1983).[7] Indeed, "*the object reveals the drives*. It does not create them – and no doubt it can be said that it is at least partly created by them – but it is the condition for their coming into existence".[8]

Furthermore, *acted on by the drives*, the Ego tends to bind itself to the object as it does to its complement. In fact, a psyche cannot by itself bind all of drive life. This is why it must bind itself to objects, whence the *binding and intertwining, therefore symbolising, function of external objects*. Thus, for the drive not to be experienced as dangerous and destructive, the subject has to be able to count on the object. Moreover, thanks to the object, the Ego succeeds in establishing within itself a regime of stable investments at a constant level.

Thus, we will say, "in the beginning was" the metapsychological couple drive/object defined by Green, the drive constituting, according to him, the *matrix of the subject*. And in light of his reflections, I can maintain that *the Ego already contains within itself a primordial couple, the metapsychological couple drive object, matrix of the future conjugal-love couple.*

The Ego's objectal environment

M. Bouvet and S. Viderman (1969)[9] consider that all the objects, both external and internal, of any subject constitute its environment, with which it organises specific relations modelled by its unconscious conflicts. They mention a continual interplay uniting the subject to its objects, – real and fantasised.

A twofold aspect is present from the beginning in Freud's work:

- The object is a constitutive element of the drive, therefore internal to the drive arrangement (source, impulse, object and goal). It is interchangeable but indispensable. There is no instinct without object.
- The object is external to the drive. It is part of the external world – perceived or represented. It is aimed at and invested by the drive in such a way that it is perceived by the subject as the cause of desire.
- It is therefore an intersection, situated both in the subject's psychic reality, organised and disorganised by the primary processes, and in external reality, outside of the subject. It is also both an object of desire and of identification.

The power of the object is only conceivable in reference to fantasy, more precisely, to the fact that the external object constitutes an *analogon of the fantasised object*, which can thus make satisfaction possible through *actualisation and realisation of the fantasy*, meaning in the enjoyment that it makes possible.

Besides, as external to the drive arrangement, the object is not at the disposal of the Ego. Consequently, the object's exteriority causes the subject's dependence on it and becomes a source of conflict.

The conflict between the Ego and the trauma-object

Indeed, the object is neither fixed nor ongoing. *It is what is unpredictable in time as well as space.* It has its own moods and desires, which only coincide partially with those of the Ego. It has its goal and its object, which are not necessarily in line with the reciprocity wanted by the Ego. Just so many *sources of traumatism*, as the Ego's inability to control it shows (Green, 1983).[10]

Conflict is then inevitable between the Ego and the trauma-object. In speaking of the *trauma-object*, Green essentially focuses on the threat that the object represents for the Ego, to the extent that it forces the Ego to modify its regime by its existence alone.

Thus, the Ego is both the seat of the effects of the trauma, but also the seat of the reactions against this dependence on the object, constituting an important part of the Ego's defences against the object, whose independent variations trigger anxiety.

Consequently, Green emphasises that the problem of relationships between Ego and object is that of limits and that of their limits, of their coexistence. These limits are just as internal as they are external, meaning that the limits between Ego and object resonate with the limits between id and Ego, something that is particularly enlightening when it comes to understanding the relationships between each conjugal partner's Ego and its love-object in particular.

Symbolising and subjectivating functions of the object

However, the object is not only a source of conflict and traumatisms. According to R. Roussillon (2008),[11] the object subjectivates or enables the subject to feel itself as such, whence the subjectivating function of the object. Through its role as protective shield in blocking arousal, its behaviours and its reverie, the object will be *object "to" symbolise*, in terms of its difference, its otherness, its absence.

But a psyche alone cannot bind all instinctual life and the "sexual" marks the limit of the intrapsychic treatment of the instinctual movements, the limit of the self-sufficiency of the individual psyche, the imperative need to bind with the objects.

This is why the psyche must bind itself to objects and find another modalities of binding. Thus, the intrapsychic opens itself up to the intersubjective through the problem of the *use of the object*, that of the external objects and their intertwining and binding, therefore symbolising functions.

This mode of using the object concerns the "object for symbolising".

Diverse representations and roles of the object that one will find with the love-object and the couple-object according to B. Brusset, 2007[12]

The object can represent an *external source of excitation* animating the subject, which represents its drives, thus triggering defences such as a protective distance. It can also be a libidinal object, partial, oral, anal or phallic, source of satisfaction.

Because it is invested by the drives (both Eros and the destruction drive), the object is perceived as dangerous, threatening or detestable (I hate it because it represents my sexuality in its raw state, I desire it, I do not love it). In contrast, the object can also play the role of protective shield.

The object can represent and play *the role of Superego* for the subject, not only as prohibitor, but as instinctual regulator and guarantor of narcissism and of the subject's autonomy, whence the paradox of a dependence on the object, which is the condition of the feeling of wholeness and autonomy.

The object can also represent and play the role of the Ego of the subject, of which it is the substitute (role of "auxiliary Ego" defined by Bouvet).[13] Thus, as "auxiliary Ego", the object will be able to help the subject, "passivised" by its instinctual motions experienced as dangerous and destructive, to make them tolerable, like a mother with her child.

The Ego's two new objects: the love-object and the couple-object

Both the love-object and the couple-object are objects, at the same time external and internal, fantasised, total and partial, objectal and narcissistic, invested by both drives, Eros and the death drive, therefore, objects of ambivalence, of love and of hate.

Just as each partner's Ego will have relations of conflictuality with these two objects, so too these objects will maintain, or will be able to maintain, conflictual relations between themselves within the Ego.

The love-object

The love-object is the love partner, another desiring subject defined as an external object, perceived and situated in external reality. It is characterised by its otherness and its autonomy, but also by the psychic work involved in its specific choice made in reference to fantasised objects of pregenital origin, primary maternal object, but also of oedipal origin, paternal and maternal objects.

This love-object will be different from the oedipal internal objects while involving partial identity bonds. It will therefore be *the product of compromise formation. Its transferential dimension* will thus update the resonance and the correspondence with the subject's oedipal, pregenital and internal objects, which are then projected onto this love-object.

Its introjection and/or its identification with it, operations of each partner's Ego's couple work, will make it an internal object that, on the one hand, will bind to the subject's internal objectal world and, on the other hand, will be able to perform several functions within the Ego, such as: source of excitation and of libidinal satisfaction; representative of the Ego's drives; function of protective shield and of drive containment; auxiliary Ego, but also, for example, a superegoic function.

Diverse relationships of conflictuality will be at work between the subject's Ego and the fantasised and internal representations of this love-object, between those representations and its perceptive, therefore external, necessarily and inevitably evolving reality.

With B. Rosenberg (1991),[14] let us examine the Eros and death drive dualism at work within this love-object – an object invested with both drives – and the effects it has on the love-object-Ego objectal relationship.

For the constitution of the "unity" of the object, for its internal binding-coherence, the libido, therefore Eros, must succeed in constituting it and preserving it – which corresponds to Green's objectalising function (1993)[15] – just as the death drive must not succeed in breaking the object apart (de-objectalising function), something that corresponds to another operation of the Ego's couple work.

To be more specific, this libido includes varied doses of objectal and narcissistic investments, as well as of homosexual and heterosexual investments.

In addition, Rosenberg maintains that a good relationship between the libido and its object, or what follows from this, between the desire and the object of the desire, necessarily involves a contribution of death drive which puts them at a bearable distance from each other, thus making an elaboration of the desire possible by avoiding direct collusion between the desire and its object.

Let us remember, moreover, that the exteriority of the love-object will be a source of traumatisms for the subject's Ego. Unlike the couple-object, it will be a *trauma-object*. From this perspective, conflict is then inevitable between the Ego and the love-object.

What about the couple-object?

Like the love-object, it will be a matter of a partially created (re-)found object. Indeed, before being a perceived living reality, the couple-object is, in the first place and historically, a fantasised internal object. I would even rather say a double fantasised object, corresponding to the infantile mnesic trace of the external parental couple on the one hand and to the still enduring fantasy of an idealised, omnipotent parental couple, *the couple-object* conceptualised by Roussillon (2008) on the other hand.[16]

These two fantasised objects are going to participate in the work of creation-construction by every subject of a couple in its living reality, which will become an external couple-object, perceived then introjected into each partner's Ego. In this way, it will become a new internal object establishing relationships of conflictuality with the external object, the living and evolving conjugal reality on the one hand and with the infantile mnesic representation of the real parental couple and the idealised couple-object on the other hand. Qualitative relationships of comparison and evaluation will be at work and generate tensions within each partner's Ego and between the two partners.

It seems to me that, unlike the love-object, the couple-object is less invested by both Eros and the death drive and that the nature of its investment is above all of a sublimated homosexual and narcissistic kind.

Both are a matter of work, that of the choice of object and that of the creation-construction of a couple, the work of Eros, of its objectalising function and of the anality of each partner's Ego.

Various kinds of relationships are at work between the love-object and the couple-object.

Apart from conflictual relationships between these two objects, an anti-traumatic and stabilising role is imaginable, – a protective shield played by the couple-object with regard to the love-object enabling the Ego to bear, in particular, the effects of this trauma-object in the manner of parents watching over and calming the child tormented by its internal and external objects.

Thus, the couple-object will introduce a triangular relationship, playing the role of a superegoic, protective, third party.

Impact of these two objects on the dynamics and economy of each partner's Ego and antagonistic relationships between couple work and individual work

While these two new objects of each partner's Ego enrich its intrapsychic and external objectal environment, having a function that is as sub-jectivising as it is binding and intertwining, therefore symbolising, they are inevitably going to destabilise its economy and its dynamic, in parti-cular the stability of its network of investments. Indeed, with the "trau-matic" encounter and the creation of these two new objects, the destabilised Ego is going to have to bear rises in the energising level that are compatible with these new "creations-acquisitions" which forces increased mastery of it and which are going to call upon its synthetic function, that is to say, its capacity to create connections among currents as a whole. These two new objects will then have to be integrated within the network of its representations replete with affects – thus instigating conflictual relationships among internal objects – and are going to stimu-late the fantasising activity, auto-eroticism and its masochism all the more.

This will be the object of highly antagonistic relations between individual work and each partner's couple work, because this new conjugal and love situation constrains the Ego to do a double job: that of adaptation and pro-tection, with its dynamic and economic components mentioned above, which is the object of the individual work, on the one hand; and that of reception, introjection and integration of its two new objects within its world of internal objects, realised then through couple work, on the other hand.

From this perspective, both the psychosexual organisation of each partner's Ego and identificatory processes for defensive purposes with regard to its two specific objects, and in particular, the love-object, the most traumatic one, will necessarily be mobilised.

The role of identification in the organisation of the defensive Ego with regard to these two objects

To the extent that the Ego is constituted in and by its relations to the object, identification becomes the essential defence against the absence of the real object and, generally, against the loss of the structuring object. Moreover, Freud mentions the role of identification as limitation of aggressiveness. It is a matter there of the projection of the subject's own narcissism who "puts itself in place of" the object and considers it as another self. Then, we can emphasise the role of inhibiting or drive contention of the Ego (Luquet, 2003).[17]

It is within the very framework of the object relation that the Ego will find the investment of possibilities of inhibiting its desires. The Ego can directly use the love-object to invest its inhibitory functions, when it will invest it as superego or as auxiliary Ego, but it can also use its relations to the oedipal imagos as prohibiting support against the use of its drives.

Indeed, each partner's Ego will be able, for example, to invest its couple-object for the purpose of inhibiting its hostile desires directed against its love-object, this couple-object resonating with its parental couple-object with prohibiting and protective functions.

The work-object, antagonistic object serving the work of the individual

Among the two conjugal partners' multiple objects of investment constituting their objectal environment, there is one that will play a major role in the economy and dynamics of each of them through the level of its sublimated homosexual and narcissistic investment, and, notably, will have a significant impact on the quality of their couple work. It is a matter of professional work and its environment, which I will call *work-object*.

One can in fact envisage the existence of competing and antagonistic relations among these three objects: the love-object, the couple-object and the work-object, something reflecting the primordial conflictuality between couple work, serving the couple's interests, and the work of the individual or individual work, serving each partner's interests.

Inasmuch as it belongs to the "world of others" within the framework of the oedipal organisation of the genital stage of the two conjugal partners (C. Parat, 1967),[18] work is an object of sublimated homosexual and narcissistic investment, a source of personal emancipation and accomplishment of a narcissistic and phallic nature, and also a source of reactivation of infantile conflicts and correlative multiple anxieties.

What is the impact of this on the partner, on the couple, on *couple work* in terms of individual and conjugal dynamics and economy?

This major object – which is a structuring sublimating path of every subject's identity that work represents and its social conditions of performing it – will maintain conflictual relationships with the two other objects, the love-object and the couple-object, to the point of being capable of considerably threatening and destabilising the subject's economic balance, as well as the economy of the conjugal and love life, consequently the economy and dynamics of each one's couple work.

Indeed, professional activity principally acts to serve individual work and conflicts with couple work.

Like the love-object and the couple-object, this work-object will be binding, intertwining, subjectivising and symbolising – an object "to" symbolise and to use "for" symbolising – just as it will also be invested by two drives, Eros and the death drive, in a different manner. The phallic and anal investments will be particularly pronounced.

However, the work-object can also play an efficacious defensive, though costly, role on the economic plane with regard to the dangers that the love-object and the couple-object represent, dangers of a narcissistic and objectal kind, in terms of dependence, invasion, intrusion and separation. Its investment of a narcissistic and homosexual kind enables each partner's Ego to establish a protective psychic distance, but it can also be a source of multiple forms of narcissistic, pregenital (sadistic – anal and phallic) satisfaction, as well as representing an outlet for destruction drives, thus partially sparing the circulation of heterodestructivity within the couple.

In addition, when this work-object is suffering, which will be a source of narcissistic wounds, an object becoming persecutory for the Ego, notably, when it reactivates the subject's paranoid-schizoid, then depressive, positions, the repercussions on the couple can be harmful on diverse accounts.

Ultimately, it is extremely important to take into consideration these three competing and essential objects of every subject's Ego and to think about their economic and dynamic impact on conjugal life and the antagonistic relationships between couple work and individual work.

Notes

1 A. Green, *Le discours vivant* (Presses universitaires de France, 1973).
2 P. Luquet, *Les identifications* (Presses universitaires de France, 2003).
3 A. Green, *Le discours vivant* (Presses universitaires de France, 1973).
4 A. Green, *Le travail du négatif* (Presses universitaires de France, 1993).
5 A. Green, *Le discours vivant* (Presses universitaires de France, 1973).
6 G. Bayle, *Clivages* (Presses universitaires de France, 2012).
7 A. Green, *Narcissisme de vie, narcissicime de mort* (Éditions de Minuit, 1983), p. 198.
8 A. Green, *Le travail du négatif* (Presses universitaires de France, 1993), p. 117.
9 M. Bouvet and S. Viderman, "La relation d'objet", in S. Nacht (ed.), *La théorie psychanalytique* (Presses universitaires de France, 1969), p. 390.
10 A. Green, *Narcissisme de vie, narcissicime de mort* (Éditions de Minuit, 1983).
11 R. Roussillon, *Le jeu et l'entre-je(u)* (Presses universitaires de France, 2008).
12 B. Brusset, *Psychanalyse du lien* (Presses universitaires de France, 2007).
13 M. Bouvet, *La relation d'objet* (Presses universitaires de France, 2006; first published 1956).
14 B. Rosenberg, *Masochisme gardien de la vie, masochisme mortifère* (Presses universitaires de France, 1991).
15 A. Green, *Le travail du négatif* (Presses universitaires de France, 1993).
16 R. Roussillon, *Le jeu et l'entre-je(u)* (Presses universitaires de France, 2008).
17 P. Luquet, *Les identifications* (Presses universitaires de France, 2003).
18 C. Parat, "L'organisation œdipienne du stade genital", *Revue française de psychanalyse*, 31, 5–6 (1967).

3 Couple work on the intersubjective level

Constitution of an intertransferential neurosis

The couple work operative at this level concerns the dynamic and the economy of the intersubjective relationship between the two partners, which itself consists of relating their systems of object relations, as well as relating their OEdipus and sibling complexes through the inter-transferential movements constitutive of an intertransferential neurosis. This couple work also consists of a *variable and flexible conjunction* of their diverse intrapsychic structural conflictualities.

We will first look at the two fundamental types of bonds with the object co-existing within every couple: the systems of object relationships and the identifications. Then, I shall return to "the oedipal organisation of the genital stage" conceptualised by Catherine Parat (1967),[1] which synthe-sises fairly well the two dimensions, dynamic and economic, of the inter-subjective relationship between the two conjugal partners, something that will help us characterise certain aspects of the couple work operative in each one.

I will continue by investigating the principal structural conflictualities animating this conjugal dynamic. This will finally lead to a disclosure of the intertransferential neurosis, which constitutes one of the essential dimensions of every conjugal organisation.

The systems of object relations

Some essential general facts

The object relation is what unites the subject to the totality of its objects. It is not the objective relation. In fact, M. Bouvet and S. Viderman (1969) consider that "any relation to real objects is modeled, adjusted in accor-dance with a primary relationship to unconscious images (fantasy object relation), hence ones affected by a coefficient of deformation which exactly measures the needs of the subject's projective defense".[2]

Consequently, the notion of object relation describes an investment of object, and therefore belongs to the domain of drives, which situates it in a continuum with the representative activity (representative-representation

DOI: 10.4324/9781003635093-6

and representative-affect). In addition, it involves twofold reference, to psychic reality on the one hand and to external reality on the other.

In their definition, Bouvet and Viderman mention the effect of the fantasised object relation on objective relations with other persons (to the extent to which they are invested as real objects), as well as a continual interplay uniting the subject to its objects – real and fantasised.

Furthermore, Bouvet (1956)[3] considers that the relational structure is the consequence of the combined action of the regression and of the fixation at pregenital stages of development.

Thus, the regressive state of the Ego or its return to archaic forms, combined with the regressive movements and fixations of drives, result in the narcissistic projection transforming the object of desire into a being similar to the subject. It is never lacking and the reality as the patient experiences it is always a transformed reality.

Following from this is the imperative necessity for any subject to establish and maintain a protective distance between it and its fantasised and real objects by *adjustments, processes of adaptation* and defensive mechanisms. However, if projection did not exist in these relationships of the subject with its important, that is to say, strongly invested objects, all these protections would obviously be useless.

For his part, in *On Private Madness* (1990),[4] A. Green identifies and describes a relationship of narcissistic identification connecting the Ego and the Other through their mutual projections. This projective current is accompanied by an introjective current, the Other feeding on projections of the Ego and inversely. The subject then never breaks free of its narcissistic projection onto object.

The object is here an object modelled on the subject's unified secondary narcissism: *the Ego and the Other are in a mutual relationship in which one is the double of the Other*, the function of the double being to be both the Same and Other.

In *The Work of the Negative* (1993),[5] Green underscores the binary structure of the relations in the Ego-Other relationship along two major lines: bisexuality (masculine-feminine) and the drive dualism through the love-hate pair.

What about relationships between transference and object relation?

Strictly speaking, transference updates interiorised systems of object relations thanks to the combined action of the regression of the Ego and of the drives with the fixation at pregenital stages of the development in the cure, as in the conjugal and love relationship.

It is at the same time a *repetition*, but also different from a pure repetition, *the creation of a new objectal relation*.

Drawing inspiration from the individual cure and its artificial production of a transferential neurosis updating the patient's infantile neurosis, we may consider that through the intertransferential movements at work between the two conjugal partners updating their interiorised systems of object relations, the couple fosters the constitution of an intertransferential neurosis, which would repeat each partner's infantile neurosis pooled together and would enable it to pursue its elaboration and /or would also foster certain points of infantile conflictual fixations.

However, a new objectal relationship would also be created between the two partners.

I will expand upon this reflection at a later point.

Economic aspects

Bouvet (1956)[6] depicts the objectal relations as a flow of drive energy, a movement controlled and adjusted by the Ego towards external objects, and he not only allows quantitative but also qualitative variations into this energy relationship. These objectal relations are both dynamically and economically necessary to every subject.

Green[7] suggests that the essential aim of the life drives is to carry out *an objectalising function*, whose role is not only to create a relationship to the object (internal and external), but also to transform structures into objects; it is also about modes of psychic activity, to the point of affirming that *it is the investment of all these activities itself that is objectalised*. This therefore leads to distinguishing the object from the objectalising function, where binding, coupled or not with unbinding, of course comes into play.

In contrast, the aim of the death drive is to accomplish, as far as possible a *de-objectalising function* through unbinding. Here, it is not only the relation to the object that is attacked, but also all its substitutes up to the *fact itself of the investment as it has undergone the process of objectalisation*. But the manifestation specific to the destructivity of the death drive is disinvestment.

For his part, B. Grunberger (1971)[8] considers that the energy approach to the objectal world is accomplished by the sensorial apparatus driven by motricity, itself the province of anality.

The energy base of any drive movement and of any objectal relationship is the anal component, and the retention factor is the basis of anal mastery and of motricity, whence the existence of an anal component in each objectal relationship. In addition, the establishment of satisfying objectal relations depends on good drive maturation, processes whose energy is also supplied by the anal component. It is anality which ensures the mastery of all the drives, anal eroticism included.

Finally, Benno Rosenberg (1991)[9] showed the role played by masochism in any object relation that it makes possible. Indeed, any object relation is a source of drive excitation. For excitation, and sexual excitation in particular, to be possible, a period of waiting-deferment, which is itself a kind of excitation and of displeasure, is necessarily obligatory. However, displeasure is only possible through masochism considered in a very broad sense as the psychism's ability to endure displeasure. It then allows relative non-satis-faction, immediate non-discharge (inherent in a lasting object relation).

It is in fact more precisely the Ego's masochistic core or primary ero-genous masochism that makes the investment (the binding) of the excita-tion possible by making it acceptable. Otherwise, excitation is unbearable (a form of displeasure) and ultimately impossible. But providing the pos-sibility of excitation, primary masochism is the guardian of psychic life. Thus, the ongoing nature of the primary masochistic core in the Ego guarantees the psychic continuity-temporality by providing the con-tinuum of the excitation.

Consequently, the assessment of the role and of the impact of the primary erogenous masochistic core at the heart of the object relation proves essential, in particular for thinking about the conditions of its durability.

Some characteristics of the genital and pregenital objectal relations

Bouvet (1956)[10] distinguishes between fundamental types of objectal rela-tions, oral and anal-sadistic, termed pregenital. We can find three kinds of objectal relations, oral, anal-sadistic and genital on this intersubjective level.

For his part, Grunberger (1971)[11] stresses, in particular, the oral-anal contrast – therefore, a *pregenitality with a dialectic dynamic.*

It seems to me to be important to present them via their diversity and singularity so as to be fully conscious of the complexity and the richness of the couple work operative within the intersubjective relationship between the two conjugal partners.

Earlier, Bouvet[12] identified an essential difference between relationships of the pregenital kind and relationships of the genital kind, which can be described from diverse points of view, as much from that of the relations between the stability of the structure of the Ego and the possession or the loss of the object as from that of the style of the relations of the subject and of the object.

Thus, specifying normality, *the genital object relation* takes into account the reality of the object, the total object, perceived in its alterity.

In this regard, Parat (1967) maintains that its development requires

> a libidinal evolution free of significant archaic fixations, flexibility in the use of defense mechanisms, an adaptability to reality and to the reality of others, a mobility of narcissistic and objectal investments, an aptitude for identifications, all of these qualities contributing to create what M. Bouvet called "the genital halo" of a personality. Reaching the genital stage goes hand in hand with sound mental structuring, which secures a certain amount of freedom with regard to the inves-ted objects, in the sense that the relational metamorphoses with these objects does not call into question the Ego's unity.[13]

As for the *pregenital subjects*, whether oral or anal, they nurture extremely close relationships with their objects, not only because such a relationship is indispensable to them, but also because the imperfect maturation of their drives compels them to do so. Fixed to a certain degree, regressive in other ways, their drives need to manifest themselves overall through violence, lack of nuance, and the absolutism of the desires and emotions of very small children.

Bouvet underscores the extreme variability of their feelings, which can be explained by their ever-present ambivalence.[14] As for the stability of their investments, it manifests itself in different ways depending on the cases. Very stable in anal-sadistic subjects, the investments appear on the contrary to display great mobility in the oral subjects. For all these subjects, the significant object is only an "object", meaning that it is only necessary to the extent that it fulfils a function, without regard for the object itself and its feelings. Owing to the regression, the positive affective tendencies have regained their destructive, aggressive "form" and the relations of the subject to the object then express all the modalities of a desire for unconditional brutal possession.

Some considerations about the identificatory work and the introjection-projection metabolism at work between the two partners

General facts

Freud defined identification as *an object relationship*. It is a matter of a relationship between subject and object, presupposing therefore a separation, joined by a movement of the libido. However, the identification eliminates this distance separating the object (perceived or represented) and the Ego.

Identification is also a *drive destiny*, retaining the object to the benefit of narcissism, which avoids seeking a new object, though at the cost of massive regression.

To the extent that the Ego is constituted in and by its relations to the object, identification becomes the essential defence against the absence of the real object and, generally, against the loss of the structuring object.

P. Luquet[15] distinguishes the identification that occurs in the total Ego or "total identification", corresponding to the "assimilation" of that which occurs in an area on the borderline of the Ego, or extension of a limited border area, corresponding to "the imagoic incorporation".

Indeed, if there is no obstacle, the incorporation is complete, and the object's function is then *taken care of* by the Ego joined to the object, which becomes a constituent of the Ego. There is a sensation of fusion with the object to the benefit of the Ego. There was *assimilation*.

In other cases, the Ego does not completely fuse with the object, which represents considerable progress when the object is perceived as dangerous. One can then speak of *inclusion* in the Ego, of object in the Ego.

These identifications are going to play a major role in the defensive organisation of each partner's Ego, whence the meaningfulness of the choice of the love-object for defensive purposes.

Some forms of identifications at work in couple work

Primary identification

For each partner, this primary identification or "joint psychic identity" (Luquet)[16] aims at being only one with the other partner in an undifferentiated fusional experience where there is no distinction between being the one or the other. It seeks to reconstitute and to relive or to live what was not able to have been lived within the mother-child unit in the state of narcissistic completeness. This primary identificatory process contributes to the structuring of every couple during the "honeymoon" phase and will contribute to sustaining the fantasy structuring its groupal reality expressed by the "we".

The projective and adhesive narcissistic identifications.

At this intersubjective level, we again find the conjunction of processes of adhesiveness through adhering to the partner, inducing a certain feeling of identity, or of continuity, and of projective identification.

G. Bayle (2012)[17] explains that it is on the parts of the partner's Ego that are the least invested in subjectivation that the union will be made with the extrusions of projective identification coming from the other partner. He underscores, in addition, that an often discreet narcissistic identity disorder of qualitative origin can ensue. It is a matter of a feeling of malaise on the part of the partner possessed by psychic elements not belonging to him or her.

One of the consequences of these two processes is a partial effacing of the psychic boundaries between the two partners.

The introjective identification

Also active are the introjective processes of identification by which the love-object is first introjected into the Ego, which will identify either with some of its characteristics or with all of them, referring to the *assimilation* of the total object defined by Luquet.[18]

Thus, at this intersubjective level, couple work accomplished by both partners would consist of processes of mutual and criss-crossed identifications, as adhesive and projective as they are introjective. As for the metabolism comprised of projections and introjections, it would be ongoing – vivifying and nurturing the conjugal economy and dynamic.

OEdipal organisation of the genital stage

It seems to me that the oedipal organisation of the genital stage elaborated by Parat (1967)[19] synthesises in a luminous way the dynamic and economic reality of every conjugal organisation termed heterosexual in its intersubjective dimension, while integrating its libidinal relationship to the "world of others", therefore extra-conjugal.

This is why I am going to recall and expand upon its principal characteristics, which will help me to explore all the better the economic and dynamic components of couple work on this intersubjective level.

It involves a twofold relation, heterosexual and homosexual, within a three-way system, composed of two conjugal partners and all "the others".

By synthesising the three components, genital, tender and pregenital into a single relationship, *the heterosexual relationship* enables a man and a woman to form *an oedipally structured couple*.

The genital component is constituted "of revived and present genital drive affects". It conditions a shared desire and genital pleasure. It is a relationship of the heterosexual kind, that is to say, in which the enhancement of the investment of the other sex is at play, the genital complementarity enabling each of the partners to live a satisfying genital relationship.

> The tender component results from the genital and sexual drives sublimated during the decline of the OEdipus complex and during the period of latency. Combined with these currents are love currents of much older pre-oedipal (ante-oedipienne) origin, the root of which can be found in the identification with a good mother image.
>
> Being able to feel him- or herself both as the child and the good mother who loved it, each conjugal partner accepts the primacy of the other's narcissism.[20]

As for the pregenital component, it involves a non-genital sexual portion of desire and of satisfaction both in a drive form, the erotic element, and in a sublimated form, the narcissistic element.

This erotic element seeks to rediscover and fulfil old fantasies and pleasures, while the narcissistic element realises an overinvestment of the love-object, which corresponds to a displacement of the narcissism itself, this love-object then finding itself mixed in with the subject's internal objects which are then projected onto the object chosen.

The homosexual relationship, which concerns all "of the others" outside the couple, is also composed of sublimated affects and of affects non-sublimated to a small extent

The elements of identification, which are very significant, mean that the others taken as a whole can be treated as "another fellow human being".

In a way parallel to the formation of a genuine interiorised Superego, after the OEdipus, all "the others" are going to drain a double libidinal current, namely:

- An aggressive, hateful current, a direct heir to the oedipal hatred, which competes to consolidate the frustrating, restrictive aspect of the investment of reality and partly conditions the efforts to adapt to society and to objective reality in general.
- An identificatory current involving superegoic projective movements, homosexual affects (for the most part sublimated), and sublimated pregenital affects, which find the opportunity to develop and be satisfied in sports, active, professional, social, etc. life.

Among "those others", who make up the society facing the couple and are not equally invested, Parat integrates: people having superegoic value, models, incarnations of an Ego Ideal, friends and children, to which I will add the professional world. She underscores on the one hand the *living, mobile* balance and, on the other hand, the *fragility* of this oedipal organisation.

I will pursue this reflection on the dynamics and the drive destinies of this conjugal libidinal organisation in Part I, Chapter 5 which is devoted to the temporality of conjugal organisations.

Structural conflictualities

These conflictualities are intrapsychic-individual and they become intersubjective when they *combine* with those of the partner. They will also animate the conjugal dynamics, and the principal aims of couple work will be, on the one hand, to make them mobile and flexible enough and, on the other hand, to avoid quantitative imbalances between the two terms of each one of them. In short, it will be a matter of creating a *game, a creative and living game*, for each one of them.

What are the conflictualities in question?

I already identified the following in *Le couple et son histoire* (2011):[21]

Eros/destruction drives, identity/otherness, narcissism/objectality, sexual identity/bisexuality, masculine/feminine, homosexuality/ heterosexuality, pregenitality/genitality, sexuality/self-preservation, Ego/love-object, Ego/couple-object, love-object/couple-object, love couple/parental couple, couple/family, private couple/public couple.

I will take a look at some of these.

Eros/destruction drives

Green (1993)[22] approaches intersubjective and intrapsychic conflictuality via the antagonism between the de-objectalising and objectalising functions I have already presented. Thus, the couple and couple work will be objectalised by the Eros of the two partners. However, through unbinding and disinvestment, the de-objectalising function of the death drive will contribute to attacking each partner's couple work, if the quantitative relationship is in its favour, leading to its failure which will manifest itself in many forms of suffering, even in a separation of the two partners and the break-up of the couple.

Identity/otherness

This conflictuality refers to the primordial and primary difference, that of the Ego and of the non-Ego, that of the "One" and of the "Other". This narcissistically unacceptable and irreducible difference will co-organise the structural conflictualities of all couples in their intersubjective dimension.

The feeling of identity is endangered in conjugal life and its identificatory work, to the extent to which, through his or her otherness, the partner, who is both object and subject, revives the basis of the subject's otherness, thus constituting a threat of identity disorganisation, while the identity is constituted on its effacement.

At the same time, the subject dimension is reinforced by the partner, and the processes of subjectivisation and symbolisation, defined by R. Roussillon (2008),[23] prove very important in conjugal functioning, because each partner is going to contribute to reinforcing the process of subjectivisation in the other, recognised as subject. However, through his or her otherness and identificatory movements, especially through projective identification, he or she is also going to threaten his or her identity.

Narcissism/objectality

Like the identity/otherness conflictuality, the narcissism/objectality antagonism occupies a central position within the dialectical relations between couple work and work of the individual.

Besides its topical and dynamic aspects, this conflictuality is particularly marked by its ongoing economic oscillations in each partner's couple work between the investments of the love-object, of the couple-object and the Ego's restorative investments.

Pregenitality/genitality

We know that pregenital elements of an oral, anal and phallic nature infiltrate and integrate themselves into the genitality of every conjugal and individual life. But genitality can also effect regressive movements towards pregenital points of fixation, which are common and shared by the two partners. These libidinal movements animate the erotic and non-erotic life of couples. The most important thing is to find an economic and dynamic balance that is mobile and flexible, but also satisfying.

However, in certain cases or certain periods of conjugal life, we can observe regressive movements on the part of one or both partners towards points of pregenital fixation which become fixed and endure to tend towards a new, predominantly pregenital, libidinal functioning.

I shall elaborate on the following conflictualities more fully: sexual identity/psychic bisexuality, masculine/feminine and heterosexuality/homosexuality.

Sexual identity/psychic bisexuality

It is essential to understand the following: on the one hand, the conflictual and indissociable connection, on both the intrapsychic level and the inter-subjective level, between sexual identity and psychic bisexuality; and, on the other hand, that the question of psychic bisexuality falls fundamentally within that of the difference between the sexes.

Let us look at psychic bisexuality first of all.

There is psychic bisexuality because there is incompleteness in each of the sexes, felt by each as castration. It is thus tied to renouncing the pleasure of the other sex and is found at the heart of the advent of the principle of reality.

Indeed, it is through the constitution of the fantasy of the other sex – the one that one does not have, but that one could imagine one has, in the oedipal triangle – that the psychic bisexuality is organised (Green, 1983).[24] And this psychic bisexuality will then integrate the difference between the sexes into the post-oedipal masculine and feminine introjective identifications.

In parallel and inversely to the differentiating evolving movement through which sexual identity asserts itself – with what that confers in terms of narcissistic reassurance and aggravation of the feeling of incompleteness – there would exist, according to C. David (1992),[25] "a bisexualizing movement", which would tend towards the interiorisation of the psychosexual difference in the form of an accentuation of the complementary schemas of the other sex that are present in each one's psyche as potentially more likely or less likely to be awake or to waking up.

Finally, psychic bisexuality is a potentiality playing a role of mediator (bisexual mediation), in particular, in the intersubjective exchanges – both sexual and psychosexual. However, it could also be an obstacle to the circulation of fantasies and investments if the complementarity it represents hypertrophies at the expense of the specific sexuality or psychosexuality tied to the actual sex, something that could have negative effects on the partner and the conjugal dynamics.

What about sexual identity or gender identity?

The core of gender identity is the conviction that the assignment of one's sex was anatomically and psychologically correct. R. Stoller (1968)[26] considers gender identity to be fundamentally grounded in the assigning of child's sex by its parents.

The more the inner certitude that the assignment of sex is firmly grounded, the more freedom the subject potentially has in expressing his or her masculine and feminine traits. Clear sexual identity in theory licenses a broad unfolding of psychic bisexuality, which is a source of psychic creativity. However, claiming real bisexuality attests to a refusal of the difference between the sexes in that it involves the absence of the other sex. It can be acted upon when sexual identity is not secure.

Within the heterosexual couple, a whole interplay will be necessary between the flexible affirmation of one's sexual identity and the use of one's bisexuality fostering changes of positions and of roles in relation to the situations of conjugal life, as well as in the identificatory processes that make it possible to offer fantasised satisfactions.

On the other hand, in certain couples, the affirmation of one's sexual identity can be an object of envy, of disparagement, just as the expression of one's bisexuality can be inhibited, even repressed, something attesting to a local failure of couple work within this conjugal organisation.

Masculine-feminine

This masculine/feminine psychosexual pair is formed during puberty and indicates a genuine difference – that of the sexes, the object of another conflict, initially intrapsychic-individual and then intersubjective, which will represent one of the major conflictualities in the course of conjugal life. The man's masculinity needs to be confirmed and reinforced by the partner, just as the woman's femininity requires confirmation from her partner, both in accordance with diverse modalities and in certain situations. However, at certain times, the woman may need to play a masculine role, just as the man might need to play a feminine role within the couple, or to invest regressively the role of a child beside a mother figure, something the woman may accept or refuse, even reject as being degrading for "her" man as well as for her, who would narcissistically overinvest the masculinity she has projected onto her partner – just as the man may reject the masculine role played by his partner who would attack his masculinity, awakening castration anxiety, in particular. Thus, many conjugal "conflicts" and reproaches are inherent in this masculine/feminine conflictuality.

I am now going to deal with some fundamental gender differences, beginning with the role of the mother as a messenger of castration for the boy and of expectation for the girl.

Let us look at J. Schaeffer's reflections (1997) on this subject. While a mother "says to the little boy who charges ahead, penis first: 'Watch out, or else you're going to have problems,' to the girl she will say: 'Wait, you will see, one day your prince will come!'".[27] However, the wait is a time of painful excitation, investment in which will mobilise the girl's primary erogenous masochism. The mother is not only going to determine the quality of her child's primary drive entanglement, but also, through her alternation of presences and absences, enable it to become organised both in fantasy, through hallucination of satisfaction, and in autoerotism. And this connection between erotism and primary erogenous masochism will play out differently in the boy from in the girl.

Thus, destined to a sexuality of conquest, meaning of penetration, the boy will most often organise himself in the activity and mastery of waiting, well-fortified by his anality and his castration anxiety.

As for the girl, her destiny is to wait. She first awaits a penis, then her breasts, her periods, she awaits penetration, then a child, then childbirth, etc. She never stops waiting. And since these unmasterable waits are for the most part connected with experiences of real losses of parts of herself or of her objects – which she cannot symbolise, as the boy can, as anxiety about losing an organ – as well as with disruptions of her narcissistic economy, she needs to be anchored in a solid primary erogenous masochism.

Let us now look at some objects of differentiated investments, such as the relationship to the body, to motricity and to language, which one encounters as difference, often conflictual, within the couple.

While the masculine is shown, displayed, bearer of the penis, and the narcissistic overinvestment of boys and men involves their penis, the feminine is hidden and the bodily erotisation is more intense. In fact, "it is their whole body that girls and women can invest as 'completely phallic,' hooked onto the reassurance of the way others look at her".[28]

However, the girls and women must speak in order to prove and at the same time hide the existence of what they have inside, just as confronting greater demands of psychic work, they must tie and verbally express more bodily experiences and affects owing to the intensity of sexual pleasure and of the transformations they feel. One can observe in them an erotisation of the vocal organs, whence the greater ease in putting their affects into words that is observable in girls and women. While, investing verbal expression much less, boys would be impelled to act to show their virility, and they would prefer to keep to the operational dimension of their conduct.

One could also differentiate between the masculine and the feminine in terms of the nature of their anxieties.

Thus, Freud[29] held that the absence of castration anxiety in girls exposes them much more to anxieties of losing everything, all being, more than all having. According to Freud, the loss of love is for the woman, the equivalent of castration in the man.

However, we find a common anxiety, namely penetration and feminine anxiety.

Schaeffer proposed to "call 'feminine anxiety' *the anxiety of penetration of the Ego and of the body by a stranger*, bearer of the nurturing breaking in of the constant drive impulse".[30]

In boys, feminine anxiety can take the form of an anxiety of homosexual penetration by the father's penis, what Freud called "refusal of the feminine". This "refusal of the feminine" by the man is both a form of defence against identification with the feminine (= castrated), and also a form of defence against the anxiety of penetrating the woman in accordance with the motricity of the constant impulse.

In girls, this feminine anxiety can constitute a "refusal of the feminine" by clinging to penis envy. But it can also be the promise of a capacity of openness to the "feminine".

> It is with regard to this anxiety for their feminine that girls and women resort to "femininity" [...], namely surface femininity [...], that of dresses, jewelry, high heels, perfumes, makeup aimed at not reflecting before men an image of a castrated woman apt to awaken their castration anxiety [...]. The emphasis is therefore placed on the visible, on the fetishist mode, in order to conceal or deny the woman's lack of a penis ... for the man.[31]

All these anxieties are reactivated within the couple, whether it is a matter of erotic life or of other areas of conjugal life.

I will stop here in order to take a look at one last conflictuality, that contrasting the two currents of libidinal investment: heterosexual and homosexual.

Heterosexuality/homosexuality

Recall that Freud (1920) considered that, alongside their obvious heterosexuality, normal individuals present a very considerable share of unconscious or latent homosexuality. Moreover, "all throughout life everyone's libido normally swings back and forth between the masculine object and the feminine object".[32]

This conflictuality inherent in bisexual desires is omnipresent in every subject and within the couple as two complementary and antagonistic modes of investment of the love-object, but also as a source of conflicts or of splitting between the heterosexual investment, prevalent and exclusive within the heterosexual couple, and the homosexual investment presumed to be exclusively directed outside the couple, as Parat (1967) maintained.[33]

There are multiple potential ways by which this universal libidinal current can infiltrate and integrate itself into both the psychosexual structure in the adult life of every subject, and into conjugal and love life. Let us look at the reflections of C. Parat, M. Fain and J. G. Lemaire.

While Parat (1967)[34] maintained that the essentially sublimated homo-sexual current of oedipal organisation is directed towards objects outside the couple with a small part investing the conjugal partner, Fain (1967)[35] considered that a couple's harmonious life makes the integration of the homosexual libido possible, extending therefore beyond bisexual forms of satisfaction.

Fain started from the fact of the narcissistic wound inherent in the negative OEdipus. Indeed, an adult facing his or her inversed oedipal conflict always revives a certain narcissistic wound and to a certain extent remains identical with the powerless oedipal child, unlike the wound fol-lowing the positive oedipal conflict, which can be healed through, among things, bodily maturation. However, in the life of a couple, one partner will offer the other partner some possibilities of identification of a hyster-ical, erotic nature and will thus represent "the potential possibility of really having sexual relations with someone of the same sex as oneself".[36] That is why he affirmed that only living as a couple can enable the inte-gration of the partners' homosexual libido. He explains, moreover, that what is most important is not satisfaction, but integration, meaning "the feeling of aptness for satisfaction involving the inclusion of the partner's sex within the limits of the Ego itself".[37]

In addition, this bond, which is both narcissistic and non-desexualised, neutralises the free aggression attached to the biological impossibility of bisexuality and is one of the rare elements conditioning a couple's union in a lasting way.

Finally, Lemaire (1979)[38] considered that a very important place must be accorded to the satisfaction of this homosexual libidinal current of each one of the partners within the couple, something that can conflict and compete with their heterosexual current.

Allow me to note that mutual co-identification and the choice of nar-cissistic object are facilitated by the importance of the homosexual current in each one of the partners.

Then, as Parat emphasised,[39] being predominant in friendly and pro-fessional relations in particular, this homosexual current will therefore foster the creation of this relational dimension of a friendly nature within the couple, thus mobilising the psychic bisexuality of the two partners, something that leads us to envisage a double, masculine and feminine, homosexual current in each partner.

Thus, the two partners of a heterosexual couple can play the role of two "buddies" or of two brothers who watch a soccer match together on television, or of two "girlfriends", even two sisters, who go shop-ping together.

Each one's feminine and masculine homosexuality will then be mobi-lised and invested in these banal situations of their daily life, something that is part of the diversity of the roles played by each one within the couple and, to the extent of the different, common and shared, dimensions of conjugal life, attesting to a psychic flexibility on the part of the two protagonists, of their couple, but also to the couple's fantasy and behavioural richness.

When this homosexual component is relatively little invested in the couple's functioning, this will translate into a poor friendly dimension between the partners, something that one sometimes observes in certain conflictual couples, where only the heterosexual component seems provisionally to maintain the couple's cohesion.

In other couples, a split would exist between each partner's two currents, homosexual and heterosexual, the heterosexual current alone defining the choice of partner and quasi-exclusively finding satisfaction in the erotic life with the partner, while the homosexual current seeks and invests objects and activities outside the partner and the couple, in particular establishing outside friendships, whence the relative psychic poverty of these conjugal organisations. Intrapsychic-individual determinants of a defensive nature would be something to explore, but also determinants of a sociocultural nature. Certain societies foster and reinforce defensive splits, in particular masculine ones.

On the defensive plane, let us look at the need certain subjects have in their relationship to the partner to be themselves unaware, or to leave the other person unaware, of the extent of their homosexual current, experienced as dangerous. So, the organisation of their heterosexual couple will have to impose a distribution of roles such that each partner is charged with confirming the partner's genuine heterosexuality and of keeping the latent homosexual current repressed but enduring, which will be satisfied outside the couple from then on.

However, the considerable extent of the permeation of the aim-inhibited current of homosexual investment within the couple can also be expressed through the two partners' little-eroticised tender attachment, which will be accompanied by a significant limitation of their erotic life (which will become somewhat secondary) and will contribute to the durability of the conjugal relationship, as Fain had found.

I will stop my reflections on this conflictuality to recall that all the conflictualities that I have brought up are interdependent and constitute a central dynamic component on this intersubjective level.

The time has now come to discuss intertransferential neurosis.

Elements for understanding the couple as an economic, dynamic and topical organisation partially constitutive of an intertransferential neurosis

Psychoanalytic practice connects transference neurosis and infantile neurosis. Indeed, within the analytic cure, M. Neyraut (1974) defines transference neurosis as "the organization of an artificial neurosis centered on the cure itself, as well as on the analyst and regrouping all the transferential manifestations".[40] S. Lebovici (1980)[41] establishes and develops the hypothesis according to which transference neurosis enables the reconstitution of the infantile neurosis, both forming a unit.

Let us follow its development, starting with the transference neurosis, followed by the infantile neurosis to arrive at Lebovici's conception of the transference neurosis-infantile neurosis unit, something that will help us conceive one of the dimensions of the conjugal organisation as intertransferential neurosis, reactivating and enabling the reconstitution of the two partners' infantile neurosis based on the work of interpreting infantile conflicts revived in the intertransference.

Transference neurosis

First, *transference neurosis* organises the patient-analyst interaction as the infantile neurosis did between the child and its family environment. Organised along conflictual lines, it is formed and blossoms within the analytic situation, on the basis of relational transferences, in particular. What are transferred are the unconscious infantile conflicts, their mode of organisation and the unconscious fantasies that can be revealed there. One will therefore be able to speak of transference neurosis to allude to an experimental situation in which the unconscious conflicts of infantile neurosis are re-expressed.

From then on, transference neurosis represents the model giving meaning to transferences and to neurotic manifestations of transference and discovers its root in the *infantile neurosis* it enables to reconstitute. Thus, it proves to be one of the effects of "afterwardness" organising the consequences of the infantile neurosis.

Infantile neurosis

As for *the infantile neurosis*, dissimulated by infantile amnesia, it can be defined as a time of organisation and as a model that will reproduce transference neurosis. If it must be situated in time, Lebovici considers that it is the translation of infantile sexuality reorganised by the phallic positions and "the tremendous investment of the penis", but also what precedes the child's possible clinical neurosis, which begins before and during the period of latency. Described as a hysterical organisation, in terms of its evolution, it translates the leap leading from the autoerotic organisation to a sexuality that is going to submit to the primacy of the genital and to the unconscious fantasy of castration, having neuroticising potentiality.

"Residue of development, process of infantile sexuality, heavy with the OEdipus complex",[42] it would be a "pre-neurosis" and the "form of the child's OEdipus complex", states Lebovici.

The afterwardness uniting the transference neurosis to infantile neurosis

It is the process of the sexualisation of the transferential relation.

> Thus, what is repeated only takes on value in the situation connected
> with the transference neurosis which summons up a past in order to
> give it meaning. There is not only superposition and adequation
> between infantile neurosis and transference neurosis. The latter
> reconstructs the former. It gives it meaning in a revelation showing
> that it is not enough to analyze technically the *hic and nunc* of trans-
> ferential relations reproducing past objectal relations. It is proper for
> these relations to take on meaning as in the past.[43]

What about the intertransferential neurosis within the couple?

Following the work of Freud, Neyraut and Lebovici, in particular, if one
considers that the couple fosters different modalities of regression in each
partner, those of the Ego as well as libidinal ones, enabling, through their
intertransferential movements, to reproduce, to update between the two,
their systems of past object relations, as well as certain infantile conflicts,
we can from then on consider that the couple constitutes an economic,
dynamic and topical organisation involving a highly pronounced dimension of intertransferential neurosis. I say "a highly pronounced dimension", because the conjugal organisation also involves new aspects that are
therefore not a matter of repetition or of intertransferential neurosis.

Thus, just as transference neurosis organises the analyst-patient interaction on the individual level, I will say that, within the couple, intertransferential neurosis contributes to organising the interactional dynamic
and economy between the two partners. It is formed and blossoms on the
basis of intertransferential movements, and what are transferred are their
infantile conflicts, their mode of organisation, their objectal relations and
the expression of their unconscious fantasies.

It will especially be a matter of oedipal conflicts – with their attendant
object relations, fantasies, affects, investments and identificatory processes in relation to the internal objects, paternal and maternal – but also
a matter of the sibling complex, with its constellation of object relations,
of affects (love, seduction, tenderness, hatred, envy, jealousy and rivalry
with a sibling figure), of investments (narcissistic and homosexual,
especially), of fantasies and of identificatory processes, of a narcissistic
nature above all.

Thus, through its dimension of intertransferential neurosis, the conjugal
organisation also constitutes a specific "experimental situation" characterised by the intertransferential revival of unconscious conflicts and
correlative objectal relations of the two partners' infantile neurosis that
they put in common. It manifests itself then through diverse clinical

expressions in the daily life of couples, certain of which will be objects of conflicts, suffering, complaints and reproaches.

However, the analysing situation with a couple will make possible and foster the expression of certain clinical aspects of its intertransferential neurosis. Their detection by the analyst and the interpretative work will enable the following: on the one hand, the reconstituting of certain fragments of each partner's infantile neurosis that they have put in common and have shared; and, on the other hand, the producing and revealing in the afterwardness of analytic work of a meaning to their conflicts and objectal relations as in the past, something that has fundamental implications for both the metapsychological understanding of the construction of couples and for the work with couples, and its benefits.

Notes

1 C. Parat, "L'organisation œdipienne du stade genital", *Revue française de psychanalyse*, 31, 5–6 (1967).
2 M. Bouvet and S. Viderman, "La relation d'objet", in S. Nacht (ed.), *La théorie psychanalytique* (Presses universitaires de France, 1969), p. 390.
3 M. Bouvet, *La relation d'objet* (Presses universitaires de France, 2006; first published 1956).
4 A. Green, *La folie privée* (Gallimard, 1990).
5 A. Green, *Le travail du négatif* (Presses universitaires de France, 1993, in French); as *The Work of the Negative* (Free Association Books, 1999, in English).
6 M. Bouvet, *La relation d'objet* (Presses universitaires de France, 2006; first published 1956).
7 A. Green, *Le travail du négatif* (Presses universitaires de France, 1993).
8 B. Grunberger, *Le narcissisme* (Payot, 1971).
9 B. Rosenberg, *Masochisme gardien de la vie, masochisme mortifère* (Presses universitaires de France, 1991).
10 M. Bouvet, *La relation d'objet* (Presses universitaires de France, 2006; first published 1956).
11 B. Grunberger, *Le narcissisme* (Payot, 1971).
12 M. Bouvet, *La relation d'objet* (Presses universitaires de France, 2006; first published 1956).
13 C. Parat, "L'organisation œdipienne du stade genital", *Revue française de psychanalyse*, 31, 5–6 (1967), p. 754.
14 M. Bouvet, *La relation d'objet* (Presses universitaires de France, 2006; first published 1956).
15 P. Luquet, *Les identifications* (Presses universitaires de France, 2003; first published 1963).
16 P. Luquet, *Les identifications* (Presses universitaires de France, 2003).
17 G. Bayle, *Clivages* (Presses universitaires de France, 2012).
18 P. Luquet, *Les identifications* (Presses universitaires de France, 2003).
19 C. Parat, "L'organisation œdipienne du stade genital", *Revue française de psychanalyse*, 31, 5–6 (1967).
20 C. Parat, "L'organisation œdipienne du stade genital", *Revue française de psychanalyse*, 31, 5–6 (1967), p. 772.
21 É. Smadja, *Le couple et son histoire* (Presses universitaires de France, 2011, in French); as *The Couple: A Pluridisciplinary Story* (Routledge, 2016, in English).
22 A. Green, *Le travail du négatif* (Presses universitaires de France, 1993).

23 R. Roussillon, *Le jeu et l'entre-je(u)* (Presses universitaires de France, 2008).
24 A. Green, *Narcissisme de vie, narcissicime de mort* (Éditions de Minuit, 1983).
25 C. David, *La bisexualité psychique* (Payot, 1992).
26 R. Stoller, *Sex and Gender: On the Development of Masculinity and Femininity* (Science House, 1968).
27 J. Schaeffer, *Le refus du féminin* (Presses universitaires de France, 2006; first published 1997), p. 172.
28 J. Schaeffer, *Le refus du féminin* (Presses universitaires de France, 2006; first published 1997), p. 68.
29 S. Freud, "The psychogenesis of a case of female homosexuality", *The Standard Edition of the Complete Psychological Works of Sigmund Freud*, XVIII (Hogarth, 1955), pp. 147–172.
30 J. Schaeffer, *Le refus du féminin* (Presses universitaires de France, 2006; first published 1997), p. 67.
31 J. Schaeffer, *Le refus du féminin* (Presses universitaires de France, 2006; first published 1997), p. 68.
32 S. Freud (1920), "The psychogenesis of a case of female homosexuality", *The Standard Edition of the Complete Psychological Works of Sigmund Freud*, XVIII (Hogarth, 1955), pp. 147–172.
33 C. Parat, "L'organisation œdipienne du stade genital", *Revue française de psychanalyse*, 31, 5–6 (1967).
34 C. Parat, "L'organisation œdipienne du stade genital", *Revue française de psychanalyse*, 31, 5–6 (1967).
35 M. Fain, "Intervention sur le rapport de C. Parat", *Revue française de psychanalyse*, 31, 5–6 (1967).
36 M. Fain, "Intervention sur le rapport de C. Parat", *Revue française de psychanalyse*, 31, 5–6 (1967), p. 822.
37 M. Fain, "Intervention sur le rapport de C. Parat", *Revue française de psychanalyse*, 31, 5–6 (1967), p. 822.
38 J.-G. Lemaire, *Le couple, sa vie, sa mort* (Payot, 1979).
39 C. Parat, "L'organisation œdipienne du stade genital", *Revue française de psychanalyse*, 31, 5–6 (1967).
40 M. Neyraut, *Le transfert* (Presses universitaires de France, 2008; first published 1974), p. 239.
41 S. Lebovici, "L'expérience du psychanalyste chez l'enfant et chez l'adulte devant le modèle de la névrose infantile et la névrose de transfert", *Revue française de psychanalyse*, 44, 5–6 (1980).
42 S. Lebovici, "L'expérience du psychanalyste chez l'enfant et chez l'adulte devant le modèle de la névrose infantile et la névrose de transfert", *Revue française de psychanalyse*, 44, 5–6 (1980), p. 819.
43 S. Lebovici, "L'expérience du psychanalyste chez l'enfant et chez l'adulte devant le modèle de la névrose infantile et la névrose de transfert", *Revue française de psychanalyse*, 44, 5–6 (1980), p. 832.

4 Couple work on the groupal level

How does one construct and keep alive a shared and common conjugal reality? I am going to explore the different aspects and modalities of it after having presented what I consider constitutes the essential elements of the very valuable contributions made by the two group analysts who have deeply inspired me: Didier Anzieu and René Kaës.

Some preliminary reflections

Invested and represented as means and locus of re-encountering the foeto-maternal fusion and later the symbiotic mother-child unit, *the experience of group*, the conjugal group in particular, is *narcissistic in nature*.

The group is in fact a figuration of an originary ensemble regressively referring to the experience of the initial caesura, that of birth and of the discontinuity between the psychic spaces of the subjects. The group and the ties producing it are, first of all, a negation of the negativity of that caesura (Kaës, 2009).[1]

In addition, *the experience of illusion* is the precondition, or rather co-extensive condition, of any tie, and at the same time it does not exist outside a tie. The groupal nature of this illusion is due to it being a common illusion, shared and maintained by the group. In order to form or to experience as a group and, as such, feel themselves mutually good or everybody to be good. (Feeling all good is a feature of this group illusion.)

Didier Anzieu and the group

Principal characteristics of groups

A group is an envelope which holds individuals together.

The groupal envelope's internal side enables the establishment of a transindividual psychic state that Anzieu (1975)[2] proposed to call a *group self*, which is imaginary and grounds the imaginary reality of groups. This groupal envelope is constituted in the very movement of the projection

DOI: 10.4324/9781003635093-7

that the individuals make of their phantasies, their imagos, their subjective topic constituted by the articulation of their psychic agencies.

Indeed, according to Anzieu, *every human group is the result of a subjective topic projected upon it by the persons making it up.* It is therefore a protean support for all the agencies of the subjective topic. For example, in real groups, projection of the Superego onto the group constitutes the most prevalent eventuality.

The group is also the container of instincts, of representative-affects and representative-representations, a place of fomentation and of sharing the phantasies and anxieties circulating among the participants.

Groups are made up of individuals and deal with the same materials and the same processes as those dealt with by the individual psychic apparatus, but this material, these processes, combine in accordance with organisations leading to productions, certain of which are specific to groupal life.

The unconscious is then grasped in the groups as a reality that is no longer intra-individual, but is inter- and trans-individual.

Economic and dynamic aspects

The group situation causes individuals to regress to schizo-paranoid and depressive positions.

In an initial phase, the group's common image is that of the *dismembered body*, then, having overcome this, the feeling of "we" arises and the group is born as a *living body* of which everyone recognises themself as a member. Having become a whole unitary body of which each member feels themself to be a part, this group represents a good object, libidinally invested, the introjected good breast.

For its members, the group also becomes a common transitional object, which for each person is both external reality and substitute, or better simulacrum, of the good breast, something bringing to the individual the presence of a neutral field, a field of the illusion, between external reality and internal reality.

While the groupal illusion enables the constitution of the group's being as a transitional object, *the breaking-apart phantasies* fulfil a unifying function by proposing to the members of a group a common denominator for personal anxieties of a different nature.

So, the antagonistic *groupal illusion–breaking-apart fantasies* pair constitutes the fundamental dialectic resiliency of the unconscious life of groups.

In addition, *in groups, as in dreams, the psychic apparatus undergoes a triple regression: temporal, topic, formal.*

The group situation in fact produces a temporal regression, not only to secondary narcissism and self-eroticism, but even to primary narcissism.

Topographically, the two main agencies of the psychic apparatus prove to be the id and the ideal Ego, which seeks to realise the fusion with the breast and the introjective restoration of this first object of love lost. For the members, the group becomes the substitute for this lost object, as I have already formulated.

As for formal regression, it is observed in the recourse to modes of expressions of the primary process, or those fairly close to it, such as figurative thought, interjections or else non-verbal manifestations such as gestures, looks, smiles, postures, mimics.

Regression is also observed in the spatiotemporal domain.

The group's imaginary space would be the projection of the mother's fantasised body, with its internal organs, including the phallus and the children-faeces.

Time also undergoes regression. It is no longer chronological, its irreversibility is abolished, leaving place sometimes for repetition and for the eternal return, at times for fantasising the return to the origins and beginning again. The spatiotemporal category proper to the group experience proves to be that of elsewhere.

Finally, while the individuals have a sex, the group does not have a sex. It is a psychic reality prior to the difference between the sexes. A natural tendency exists in each group to even out any sexual differences among its members.

We are dealing with the *narcissistic identifications* of the members among themselves with their fusional participation in the omnipotent and self-sufficient breast of the mother, who is experienced as a partial object.

Consequently, the unconscious sublimated homosexual, narcissistic investments are stronger there and have the advantage of constituting a good defence against potential aggressiveness among the members. In addition, the individuals ask for *basic narcissistic security* from the natural groups to which they belong.

Distinguishing two levels, that of structure, that of organisation

A psychic agency common to the individual apparatuses is going to structure a *groupal apparatus* which makes the production of fantasised organisations possible.

In fact, this groupal psychic apparatus is a construction that operates through a double propping up: on the one hand, on the individual psychic apparatus components; on the other hand, on the surrounding culture and the collective representations it produces and conveys.

This dominant, common agency will thus serve as an envelope, as "Skin-Ego", for the groupal psychic apparatus, thus ensuring its unity, its continuity, its wholeness, its peripheral differentiation between inside and outside.

Depending on the nature of this groupal apparatus, the group's conscious and unconscious psychic functioning will be different, with impact on the group's conduct with respect to its objectives and to external reality.

Thus, the Superego of one of a group's participants can resonate, be in collusion with the Superego of the other members. By imposing norms and rules, the group will contribute to the satisfaction of each person's superegoic demands and expectations and will find its cohesiveness in guilt feelings.

The group can also try to find a common id as an envelope for itself. Depending on the nature of the dominant drive or depending on its stage of evolution, varied collective phenomena may manifest themselves there.

In addition, suffering from the lack of a real body, *the groupal psychic apparatus seeks to endow itself with an imaginary body.* So, the metaphors of the group as "body" and of the individuals composing it as "members" aim, among other things, at realising this desire of the *group self* to take up residence in a living organism.

This topical arrangement structuring the groupal apparatus essentially manifests itself in the form of a fantasising circulation among the members of the group.

What does it consist of?

Anzieu reminds us that the relationships among human beings organise themselves around two major poles, fantasised and technical, which amounts to saying primary and secondary processes.

If the technical pole connected with the development of the conscious-ness-perception system and with the accomplishment of common tasks enables the circulation of goods and ideas, the unconscious interhuman bond – in the couple, in the group, in social and family life – results from *fantasising circulation.*

Indeed, as soon as there is a group, *a fantasising activity circulates among the members owing to the direct communication of their unconsciouses.* It con-nects them, both in their active cohesiveness and in their collective anxiety. Anxiety in face of a predominant fantasising activity causes its paralysis, while the disparity of their fantasies can cause disunion in the group. The convergence of fantasies and their unifying elaboration can either give birth to an ideology, even to a mythology, both defensive and proper to that group, or place the energy to carry out its activities at its disposal.

Thus, all human activity aiming to satisfy the needs of the organism or of the social body brings into play a fantasising dimension that stimulates, re-orients or prohibits real technical achievements.

Five unconscious psychic organisers of groups

The individual fantasy

The *fantasising* activity in the individual psychic apparatus is particularly stimulated among two or three persons by love or profound friendship.

In a certain groupal situation, certain members at times serve as identi-ficatory points of reference for others and at times as projective supports for their subjective topic and their drives, which would be the basis of the possibility of the phenomenon of the *fantasising resonance,* which is the regrouping of certain participants around one of them who, through their acts, way of being or remarks showed or made understood one of their unconscious individual fantasies.

According to Anzieu, the other members unconsciously delegate to that person the difficult and necessary dual function of forming compromises among the id, the Superego and the reality. They unload taking responsibility for the conflicts of their individual psychic apparatuses onto the groupal apparatus. The individual rightly qualified as central is then placed in the position of being the group's Ego. The leader is an arbitrator.

The imago

The imago emerges as the group's obvious organiser when the latent structure of the groupal apparatus is marked by the predominance of one of the agencies of the individual psychic apparatus: the Ego's ideal, ideal Ego, Superego. Anzieu considers that the imago confers greater stability upon the group, the group with an imagoic foundation being able to survive a change of leaders more easily than the group organised around the fantasy of an individual.

The originary fantasies

Here are some examples of these originary fantasies in group situations:

- The intra-uterine fantasy would thus be represented by the group's imaginary space and the symbolic exploration of the image of the interior of the mother's body.
- The fantasy of seduction would be activated by the forms of pairing within the group.
- The fantasy of the primal scene would come up in the triadic situation which allows for all the possible permutations of this fantasy.
- The castration fantasy would be found in the breaking-apart phantasies associating phallic castration anxiety and oral anxiety of separation from the breast with, for example, the themes of infirmity, of impotence.

As Anzieu sees it, this third organiser seems to be the one most specific to informal groups, whether small or large.

The OEdipus complex

The psychic envelope of the groupal apparatus

These five organisers present in all groups are independent regarding their nature and interdependent regarding their functioning. Generally, one of them prevails, but the repressed, antagonistic or complementary role of the others must be identified.

Principles of the psychic functioning of the groupal apparatus

Anzieu considers that, to the extent that it is not identical with the individual imaginary, the groupal imaginary proceeds from three principles of psychic functioning relating to the groupal apparatus.

- *A principle of indifferentiation between the individual and the group* (tendency towards isomorphy) makes the group tend towards an *external individuality* – through which it distinguishes itself from other groups.
- *A principle of the group's self-sufficiency in relation to social and physical reality.*
- *A principle of delimitation between an inside and an outside of the group.*

René Kaës, the model of the groupal psychic apparatus and the unconscious alliances

The groupal psychic apparatus

Kaës (2015)[3] holds that the group is the locus of the overlapping conjunction of three spaces of psychic reality: that of the group as specific entity; that of the intersubjective bonds that form there; and that of the singular subject, inasmuch as it is a member of the group and initially constituted as subject of the group.[4]

Unlike the model proposed by Anzieu, Kaës' model of the groupal psychic apparatus does not only describe the psychic space proper to the group, but also each of the three spaces of the psychic reality of which the group is composed. It is not an extrapolation of the individual psychic apparatus, but possesses its own organisation and its own functioning.

Thus, Kaës characterises the group's psychic space as being what is "common" and "shared", as defined in the following way:

> What is common is the psychic substance uniting the members of an ensemble, no matter what the configuration may be: a family, a couple or a group. Common or becoming common are: a fantasy, a dream, a desire, identifications, ideals, signifiers, an illusion, unconscious alliances. It requires the abandonment or loss of the subjects' individual limits in the bond, a certain indifferentiation, but is also the basic psychic matter necessary for the emergence of the subject in their singularity. There is no bond of group, of family, of couple without these formations and these common psychic processes.

Kaës names some of them: group culture and mentality, the groupal matrix, the groupal illusion, the unconscious alliances, the groupal associative chains, the shared and common dream spaces and fantasies, etc.[5]

For its part, what is "shared" corresponds to the share each subject takes, or to the unique and complementary place occupied in a fantasy, an alliance, a contract, a defence system common to those subject to a tie.[6]

This apparatus performs specific work, the function of which is to bind, tune, arrange and transform certain formations and certain processes coming from the psychic spaces of the subjects who become members of the group by means of this work. Kaës explains that it is a structure independent of the psyches that it assembles in a combinatory arrangement in keeping with its own laws, but it is also a construction interiorised by the members of the group.[7]

The groupal psychic apparatus is the structure and the process presiding over the specific tuning of the internal groups of the members of the group and over the arrangement of their topic, their economy and their psychic dynamics.

What are these internal groups?

They are not only unconscious internal objects, but configurations of objects, systems of objects associated by internal bonds. They display a general property of psychic matter, that of psychic groupality, namely that of being able to be associated or dissociated, incorporated or separated, whence Kaës' idea that the Unconscious and the psychic space are first of all structured as a group.

He distinguishes between two categories of internal groups:

- Originary psychic groups and their offshoots, such as the originary fantasies, the oedipal and sibling complexes, the body images, the "inter-agency" relationships of the second topic.
- The psychic groups constructed by the introjection of primary ties and the configurations of internal objects obtained by the different modalities of the identifications, in particular, by the introjection of the interpersonal relations: the internal family, for example.

This arrangement of the psyches of the members of a group demands some psychic work, arrangement processes, sociocultural and psychic organisers. Finally, it involves three poles:

- The isomorphic pole corresponds to the formation of a common, indifferentiated psychic space. There is, therefore, identity of the groupal psychic space and the individual psychic space.
- The homeomorphic pole is characterised by the differentiation between the individual spaces and that of the group, between the internal group and the external group, but also among the subjects themselves who are members of the group.
- An unstable field oscillates between these two poles as the result of the chaotic instability of the tuning of the psyches.

Finally, this model of the groupal psychic apparatus describes the psychic work of creating, maintaining and transforming processes, functions and psychic formations common to members of the group.[8]

The notion of unconscious alliance

Whatever their foundation, their function and their purpose may be, Kaës (2009) maintains that "the unconscious alliances realise the ties, all the ties, intersubjective, transsubjective and social, both those connecting the generations to one another and those connecting contemporaries to one another".[9] They are transmitted from one generation to another, with or without transformation, and produce their effects beyond the subjects, circumstances and the time that generated them.

He considers that:

> in all the configurations of linking – groups and families, couples and institutions – the unconscious alliances are concluded through a sealing of the unconsciouses of the subjects tuned to produce them. It is upon such alliances that the psychic reality in the ties and, in part, the unconscious psychic reality of the subjects of the tie are shaped.[10]

However, to constitute themselves and remain stable, they impose *psychic work* on its subjects, which will especially involve identificatory processes, drive investments, the bringing into play of unconscious fantasies as organisers of the tie, and also diverse kinds of defensive operations.

He identifies four major types of unconscious alliances.

(1) The *structuring alliances*, both *primary*, such as the *narcissistic contract*, and *secondary*, whose functions are necessary for the structuring of every subject's psyche.

The *narcissistic contract* organises the terms of a *narcissistic exchange*. It prescribes, for any subject, from the time of birth, a place within a group becoming *the group to which the subject belongs* provided that they contribute to its continuity and preservation. This *narcissistic contract* ensures both the group's growth and the conditions necessary for the narcissistic anchoring of the subject's psychic life.

(2) As for the *secondary structuring alliances*, Kaës finds in Freud's work three forms of alliances whose function is doubly structuring, both for the subject considered in their singularity and for the cultural and social institutions: *the Brothers' pact, the alliance with the Father* and *the contract of renunciation of the direct satisfaction of destructive drive aims*.

They are characterised by the relationship that they maintain with common law and fundamental prohibitions – the triple prohibition of incest, cannibalism and murder – and are thus concluded between subjects and a group, which imposes on them as a condition of social life and of their belonging to a community.

Within this dual function, these alliances play a role of symbolic guarantor and third party, generators of processes of symbolisation.

(3) *The defensive unconscious alliances and denegative pacts* and their potentially alienating and pathogenic effects form a third type of alliance.

The group – and more generally any configuration of ties – is not only the means and locus of the satisfaction of individual unconscious desires, but it is also the means and locus of the experience of hatred, of destruction, of death, of the unthinkable. In other words, the subjects also establish their ties on the basis of what they reject or deny.

So it is that with the category of the *negative,* the tie and the alliance can also be thinkable in the dimension of castration, of what is lacking or what is lost, or of what defies death. Consequently, through its diverse figures, *this negativity must be repressed, or denied, rejected and effaced.*

For Kaës, the denegative pact, which is a pact about the negative refers to "the result of the production work of the unconscious, which is necessary for forming and maintaining the intersubjective tie when the subjects of this tie are mobilised by different figures and modalities of the negative".[11]

Thus, the denegative pact will deal with negativity, either by denying it, or by linking it in an unconscious alliance said to be defensive in its subjects. Specifically concluded to ensure the defensive needs of the subjects linked, it therefore exercises a metadefensive function for each of them and will have to be envisaged as a modality of resolution of intrapsychic conflicts and groupal or intersubjective conflicts.

When the denegative pact is built on the repression and renunciation of the direct satisfaction of destructive drive aims, repressed contents result that are always in a position to return in the tie in the form of neurotically structured shared symptoms.

However, *when it establishes itself on the basis of denial, rejection and disavowal,* it creates something enigmatic, unsignifiable, untransformable in the tie and in each one of its subjects. Effacements, zones of silence, "spaces for rubbish" keep subjects strangers to their own life story and that of the other person. It is a matter of what are called *alienating* alliances which run up against the repressing function of subjects linked there.

(4) Finally, *the offensive alliances* are concluded in order to impose a creative or destructive project.

All these alliances differ from one another in their principal object and in their aim. Moreover, these alliances imply a complementarity and synergy among the subjects concluding them, whence the existence of heterogeneous and homogeneous, symmetrical and asymmetrical alliances

How is one to conceive the modalities and productions of couple work on this groupal level on the basis of these essential insights?

Going back to certain of Anzieu's and Kaës' ideas and proposals, I will respond by saying that, as a group, the couple would first be an *envelope* that holds the two partners together, but also a *container* of their drives, representations and affects, a place of fomentation, of sharing and of circulation of their fantasies and anxieties.

The couple can also conceive of itself as being an intermediate object, defining a new reality, a transitional, intermediate area, a zone of overlap between two individual areas, that of each partner.

Economically speaking, whether the couples are hetero- or homosexual, their groupal psychic reality will also be asexual, grounded in homosexual and narcissistic investments, whence another destiny, conjugal in this case, of each partner's homosexual libidinal current. The primary and narcissistic identifications will also be predominant there.

On the dynamic level, we can find the triple regression (temporal, topic and formal) of the psychic apparatus of each partner in the couple, as well as that called spatiotemporal.

In addition, we easily find the two dimensions identified by Anzieu: the fantasising circulation between the two partners (the expression of the primary process) and the technical pole, connected with the carrying out of their common tasks (the expression of the secondary process of the two partners' Ego). In this way, they form a *work couple.*

The convergence of these two dimensions will give birth, in particular, to the production of a *conjugal culture* constitutive of a *conjugal identity* realised through the two partners' joint couple work that will become, at this level, the work of their conjugal psychic apparatus. Let us recall the principal characteristics.

"Living together" presupposes the creation of a shared, common spacetime that will inevitably be in a state of tension with the partners' separate, differentiated space-times. It is a matter of fields of fomentation and of flow of fantasies, of multiple symbolisations and sublimations, within which the forming of conjugal and individual compromises will be worked out, which will find expression:

- through the creation and investment of shared and common, as well as separate and differing (professional, extraprofessional, leisure) activities;
- through the elaboration of common and unshared representations and ideas (those of men and of women, of their respective roles within the couple, of their relationships within the couple, those of the couple, inspired by their respective families, those of the family, in particular);
- through the establishment of stable and variable forms of communication, of norms of conduct, of rules of household organisation and

functioning – of common ideals and values, of mythical tales, of ritual activities evolving into habits, erotic life also figuring among them;
• through the establishment of institutions said to be "conjugal".

We can also envisage the organisation of a household economy involving incomes, expenditures, a common and differentiated budget, and also differentiated areas and ways of exercising power between the two partners. Also to be mentioned are the interplay of investments within the couple, their sphere of intimacy, its boundaries and the external world, the relationships between the private couple/public couple and their possible splitting. Finally, there is the investment of non-shared and shared time – their common and individual (past, present, future) temporality are also significant and virtually conflictual areas of any conjugal life.

Regarding psychic organisers, can we identify certain of them, or all of those mentioned by Anzieu?

We can in fact easily find individual fantasies and the correlative fantasising resonance, originary fantasies, the OEdipus complex, as well as the imagos. We will come across them again within the internal groups conceptualised by Kaës.

What about the conjugal psychic apparatus?

I will pursue Kaës' relevant approach, which corresponds to my representation of the psychic reality of couples involving three levels or psychic spaces.

This will enable us to envisage *the existence of a conjugal psychic apparatus that proves to be a specific production of both partners' couple work on this group level*. Both a structure and a process, this conjugal apparatus performs a specific form of work whose function here is to tie, to *conjoin* certain formations and processes that come from and belong to the psychic reality of the two partners who become members of their conjugal group by means of this couple work. Just as it performs the arrangement of their psychic topic, economy and dynamics.

It will remain active in each partners' psyche in order to contribute to unifying the three group, intersubjective and individual levels.

However, suffering from the lack of a real body, *the conjugal psychic apparatus seeks to endow itself with an imaginary body*.

Do not people say, or do not we hear: "we are fine *in* our couple" or, on the contrary, "things don't feel right, there's no breathing space, it's stifling, there a feeling of being imprisoned ...". The couple is, in fact, experienced as being fantasised by its two members, not only as a "living body", but also invested as a growing living being with functional, psychic and vital needs to satisfy, which inevitably goes through critical periods of change and maturation.

However, this representation of a living being, of a "living body" different in the two members will arouse or will be able to arouse varied fantasies generating diverse, essentially archaic, anxieties of being devoured, swallowed up or persecuted, for example.

This fantasy of a *unitary, living body and of being alive* is antagonistic to the representation of the *dismembered body and of the suffering living being* emerging in a period of crisis, animated then by breaking-apart fantasies, accompanying the reactivation of the two partners' paranoid-schizoid and depressive positions.

The conjugal group or couple-object, a fantasised living being and a shared and common creation, though differentiated in each of the partners in the double form – perceived and represented – then seems to me to represent a third psychic object within the intersubjective love relationship, which therefore proves to be triangular. This conjugal group or couple-object receives an investment of a narcissistic and homosexual nature.

This conjugal psychic reality also rests on a set of unconscious alliances that are structuring, but also defensive and offensive. It is a matter of another type of production of couple work.

The conjugal narcissistic contract

First, let us look at the *conjugal narcissistic contract* existing in every couple.

It is a matter of a *contract of affiliation* to the couple as a secondary group that receives and requires from each partner both sublimated homosexual and narcissistic investments in the service of the self-preservation of the couple and of each of its members.

It prescribes a place for each person within the couple providing that they contribute to its continuity, its preservation and its evolution. In addition, an Ego Ideal and shared and common objects are going to be created by extracting a portion of narcissism from each one – in particular, the conjugal identity and culture with all their diversity.

This conjugal Ego Ideal will exercise a repressive function on each of the members of the couple and will oblige them to respect the terms of their contract in the name of their conjugal Ideal. However, every time there is a reorganisation of the narcissistic foundations of the conjugal bond, a gap can occur in relation to the initial narcissistic contract, which will be accompanied by a return of what has been repressed allowing the emergence of conflicts between the narcissistic demands of each person's Ego and those of the couple.

Conjugal ruptures are also ruptures of the initial narcissistic contract engendering pain, disillusionment, betrayal and mourning work.

Complementing the *conjugal narcissistic contract, the secondary structuring alliances* (the Brothers' pact, alliance with the Father and contract of renouncing the satisfaction of destructive drive aims) represent metapsychic guarantors also constitutive of the conjugal space with its fundamental prohibitions.

What about defensive alliances?

Within the couple, different defensive operations are required of each partner for the bond to be able to be constituted and maintained, at the risk of its destruction. Thus, a joint treatment of the individual defence mechanisms and of the defence mechanisms proper to the conjugal bond will be at work to the benefit of its partners and to that of their couple.

When the conjugal denegative pact is built upon repression, repressed contents result that return by way of transference, symptoms of a neurotic nature, dreams, slips of the tongue. Their structure is that of compromise formation sustained by a metadefence, the function and purpose of which is to subject each partner to their symptom in relation to what they achieve in and for the conjugal bond. We must then take into consideration, on the one hand, the value and dual individual function – economic and dynamic – that the symptom fulfils for the partner themself, and, on the other hand, its value and its dual conjugal function, because this symptom also receives an investment on the part of the other in order to hold the conjugal bond together.

However, it may happen that only one of the two partners of the alliance chooses to represent it, apparently sparing the other from having to exhibit it. That partner becomes the couple's *symptom-bearer* for reasons concerning them individually of which they both make use. This is their *phoric function*.

When the denegative pacts are established on the basis of denial, rejection and disavowal, they produce unconscious contents in the conjugal bond and in each partner, which manifest themselves in acting out, massive projections, splittings, rejections, enigmatic or crude signifiers of a kind that usually remain encysted in the common denials and the perverse contracts.

Beatrice, 40 years old and Marc, 43 years old, are married and have lived together for 15 years. They are the parents of two girls, 12 and 10 years old.

They have already suffered from the loss of their conjugal erotic life for several years. In fact, it never really existed and seemed particularly unsatisfactory for each of them, Marc being a "premature ejaculator" and Beatrice not knowing how to seduce and reassure him. In addition, I learn that their communication, both verbal and affective, is very poor, essentially taking place on a factual level.

In the course of our work together, I was to discover that they were both unwanted children. When young, Marc felt excluded from the parental couple very early, disturbing their intimacy and intruding into their "fusional-symbiotic bubble", something that produced deep narcissistic wounds in him and early affective privations, as well as intense hostile impulses, especially directed towards his mother, as his father seemed more receptive towards him. However, his particularly pronounced castration anxiety kept him from confronting his father. In addition, his mother did not attach much importance to the development of his virility.

For her part, feeling she was one girl too many in her family, Beatrice grew up with the implicit obligation not to disturb her parents, not even to manifest her existence to them, to the point of developing what is called a "fusional" relationship with her mother and even of effacing any expression of femininity. She behaved then as a "tomboy", something that suited everyone, *in theory*.

Marc and Beatrice came together, then, around a shared and common set of problems – on the one hand, narcissistic wounds and early affective privations that were still alive, and, on the other hand, a rejection of Marc's masculinity and Beatrice's femininity. They also share the anxio-genic presence of an unconscious incestuous fantasy, accompanied by common defences mobilised to protect themselves from it. Something manifested, in particular, by the sacrifice of their conjugal sexuality that became the terrain of a reactivation of their childhood narcissistic wounds.

Marc's lack of erotic interest in his wife as well as the lack of appreciation of her femininity was reactivating narcissistic wounds in her. It was colliding with Beatrice's mother's rejection of her femininity, but was protecting her from the satisfaction of her unconscious incestuous fantasy with the father of her childhood, whom she, unlike certain of her sisters, did not succeed in seducing.

Marc's lack of interest in his wife also signified punishment in Beatrice's unconscious imagination, relieving an unconscious feeling of guilt connected with her incestuous fantasy.

During all those years, Beatrice had settled into a state of waiting and passivity with regard to Marc, demonstrating a quite pronounced masochistic disposition. In this way, she indirectly rejected Marc's dormant virility. He was finally able to verbalise that the sexual act was disgusting and had a destructive aggressive dimension, something underlain by an unconscious incestuous fantasy heavily charged with hostility towards the mother of his childhood, whom Beatrice represented transferentially.

They had both made a denegative pact based on the repression of the incestuous fantasy and on an unconscious feeling of guilt, which was expressed by a need for punishment. Marc was unconsciously designated by each of the two partners and by the couple to be the conjugal symptom-bearer. In this way, Marc's symptom fulfilled a double function, dynamic and economic, individual and conjugal, as well as being invested sadomasochistically by him, Beatrice and the couple. For Marc and Beatrice, the absence of conjugal sexuality was constituting a "conjugal neurotic formation", meaning a solution that was both a defensive solution, because it was protecting them in this way from their unconscious incestuous fantasies, and a sadomasochistic, punitive solution, because it was reactivating their childhood narcissistic wounds awaiting treatment.

Having come to the end of this development of ideas, I believe that with Anzieu and Kaës, I have sufficiently explored the conjugal-groupal reality and the diverse modalities and productions of couple work in its relationships with the conjugal psychic apparatus – another example of the extreme complexity of the tridimensional conjugal psychic reality.

Now, I will look at the couple through its psychic temporality, its determinants and its vicissitudes.

Notes

1 R. Kaës, *Les alliances inconscientes* (Dunod, 2009).
2 D. Anzieu, *Le groupe et l'inconscient* (Dunod, 1984; first published 1975); as *The Group and the Unconscious* (Routledge, 2014).
3 R. Kaës, *L'extension de la psychanalyse* (Dunod, 2015).
4 R. Kaës, *L'extension de la psychanalyse* (Dunod, 2015), p. viii.
5 R. Kaës, *L'extension de la psychanalyse* (Dunod, 2015), p. 69.
6 R. Kaës, *L'extension de la psychanalyse* (Dunod, 2015).
7 R. Kaës, *L'extension de la psychanalyse* (Dunod, 2015), p. 126.
8 R. Kaës, *L'extension de la psychanalyse* (Dunod, 2015), p. 138.
9 R. Kaës, *Les alliances inconscientes* (Dunod, 2009), p. 4.
10 R. Kaës, *Les alliances inconscientes* (Dunod, 2009), p. 36.
11 R. Kaës, *Les alliances inconscientes* (Dunod, 2009), p. 113.

5 Couple work and temporality

How is one to approach the temporality of the couple and of its two members? What role does each partner's couple work play in the construction and the experience of this conjugal temporality? How will the drive investments of each partner and of the couple be distributed among these different time periods, past, present and future? Conflicts will inevitably arise in accordance with the periods of life, critical stages of each partner, and also with the critical periods that the couple goes through.

Recall the three dimensions of the couple – sexual-bodily, sociocultural and psychic – each one of which necessarily has its own temporality. Conflictual relations having multiple repercussions will then be inevitable, on the topic as well as on the dynamic and economic planes. However, while aware of the interrelations among these three dimensions, here I am looking at the temporality of its psychic reality.

So it is that I discuss some dynamic and economic aspects of conjugal temporality, in particular its critical essence, to be differentiated from the "conjugal crisis". Then I enquire into certain evolving perspectives, without expanding upon the question of the ageing of the two partners and its impact upon conjugal functioning (which I addressed in *The Couple: A Pluridisciplinary Story*).[1] I continue by examining some essential conditions of the durability of a psychically living couple. Finally, I raise some questions and propose some elements of responses regarding the issues involved in the separation of the two partners and the conjugal break-up.

Economic and dynamic aspects of the couple's evolution

The couple is a living economic, dynamic and topic organisation, that is to say mobile and evolving, the apparent stability of which is determined both by relationships of force pertaining to the economy of the drive intertwining between Eros and the death drive and by recurrent processes of disorganisation and reorganisation.

Its temporality is animated by progressive movements and regressive movements towards points of pregenital fixation but also by diverse forms of repetition compulsion and afterwardness.

DOI: 10.4324/9781003635093-8

Thus, we can find a compulsion to repeat situations of pursuit of a previously repressed pleasure, a compulsion in accordance with the pleasure principle, as well as a compulsion to discharge by action corresponding to a compulsion in accordance with the Nirvana principle, then a compulsion to replay the traumatisms beyond the pleasure principle.

C. Parat (1967)[2] considers that the oedipal organisation to which the couple corresponds involves a situation "of mobile equilibrium in perpetual rearrangement", the economy of which proceeds from the living interplay of the two varieties of investments – heterosexual and homosexual – which are themselves mobile. "A sort of balancing exists between the relative importance of the investment of the one and of the other, and it is this ongoing oscillation which makes balancing it possible".[3]

This living and moving equilibrium separates the conjugal relationship from the essential part of the aggressive drives, which are found diverted towards the outside in investments aimed at the "world of others" in a very often sublimating manner.

From another, systemic and psychoanalytic, point of view, J.-G. Lemaire (1979)[4] considers that the apparent stability of couples can be understood within the framework of a dynamic balance resulting from a constant reorganisation of the interrelations between the partners, that is to say, consisting of processes of organisation, of disorganisation and of reorganisation. The couple must then be considered functionally as a whole punctuated by alternations of phases during which phenomena of honeymoon and crisis reappear in a minor form and tangled up with one another.

By permitting the affective reinvestment of the outside world, which had been partially disinvested when the partner and the couple were overinvested, crisis represents the antithesis of the honeymoon phase. In this way, the manifestations of mutual aggressiveness that the honeymoon phase had reduced and diverted towards the outside world reappear.

From then on, the conjugal evolution depends on the balance of the forces of binding and unbinding that every couple achieves.

In considering the two poles of the psychic existence constituted by organisation and stability, on the one hand, and historicity, on the other, B. Rosenberg[5] (1991) offers us a drive understanding of the evolving dynamic of the couples based on the economy of the drive intertwining.

Eros and the death drive in fact conflict through opposite *movements* of signification (integration-disintegration) and direction (regressive-progressive). So, Rosenberg considers that the drive direction of the psychic organisations involves two primary and fundamental characteristics: a first, *anti-regressive* one, which consists of the fact that every organisation strives to resist the disintegrating, therefore regressive, movement of the death drive, while the second, *progressive*, characteristic, consists of the fact that every organisation is capable of transforming itself in order to serve in this way as a constituent of larger organisations, thus making possible the progressive movement deriving from the work of Eros.

These two characteristics can come into conflict insofar as an anti-regressive, defensively oriented organisation rigidifies in order to resist the disintegrating movement of the death drive by actually losing the capacity to transform itself, thus reducing its progressive nature.

Within the internal economy of the life drive, there is therefore a whole interplay of balancing going on between the libido that works hard to defend/preserve the objectal positions acquired, and the libido that is free to invest new objects and to constitute new organisations around them.

In this respect, the fixations act – owing to this specific attachment to the object – to attract repression, and especially regression, and constitute a barrier preventing a yet greater and more profound regression. From the point of view of the drive direction, they thus represent a reinforcement of the anti-regressive nature of certain organisations by an overinvestment of Eros, which prevents their dissolution by thus checking their regressive movement.

Consequently, the internal economy of the life drive brings either its anti-regressive characteristic (self-preserving-Eros) or its progressive characteristic (libido-Eros making the objectal relations evolve) to prevail. However, this internal economy of the life drive is subject to the economy of the drive intertwining, that is to say, to the respective force, at a given time, of the life drive in relation to the death drive. It is at the heart of the object, as I have already mentioned, and of psychic organisations, and, according to Rosenberg, would constitute the ultimate factor determining the stability and the continuity of the psychic organisations, something observable on this intersubjective level of every conjugal organisation, where the movements of this economy of the drive intertwining will determine its stability or its instability and its diverse fates, among which are the separation of the two partners and correlative destruction of the couple.

The couple's critical essence and the conjugal crisis

For my part, on the dynamic plane, I distinguish between the critical essence of the couple and the conjugal crisis. I, in fact, situate the couple within the dynamic of its "natural life cycle" marked by conjugal and individual critical trials and stages that will represent situations and events, both happy and painful, existential changes, objects of necessary mourning work. They will inevitably destabilise, even upset, each partner's and the couple's psychic economy, as well as reactivating, even exacerbating, intra- and intersubjective structural conflictualities, narcissistic wounds, traumatic experiences and multiple anxieties of an oedipal and pregenital nature. They will also reactivate or exacerbate an unconscious feeling of guilt, hatred, movements of envy and jealousy up until then thought to be mastered and contained in the intrapsychic space and/ or the intersubjective space. On the other hand, they will also be able to satisfy desires for accomplishment, narcissistic completeness and even fantasies of omnipotence.

With respect to this, what is meant by "couple crisis", a usual and banal expression that everybody uses?

Couples ordinarily speak of "crisis" to convey that things are no longer going well between the two partners, when their conjugal life is neither serene, nor tranquil, but rather animated by somewhat painful fluctuations.

While they present the conflicts to us as episodic, occasional fiery outbursts that lead to a resolution of the crisis or resolve it (even if they reoccur with variable frequency and play out in rather ritualised scenarios), the conjugal crisis is experienced and described as an anguishing, conflictual and painful state, which lasts and marks a more or less sudden break in the continuity of conjugal life. The partners often experience it as an abnormal phenomenon, even at worst, as a war, although they are conscious that every couple inevitably goes through similar stages and critical times. Moreover, is it a matter of an individual crisis experienced by one of the two that has critical repercussions on the couple, or of a conjugal crisis correlative to a conjugal event, even of a family crisis having an impact on the parental couple?

André Ruffiot[6] (1984) considers that the conjugal crisis establishes a psychic kind of functioning within the couple that presents all the psychotic virtualities involving processes of denial and splitting of both the love-object and the Ego into good and bad, which are associated with a paranoid experience of the introjected partner, who from then on has become a bad love-object, an internal persecutor endangering the Ego's psychic integrity. This suggests that the conjugal crisis may reactivate the paranoid-schizoid position in each partner and within the couple, while it will be resolved through an evolution towards a depressive position implementing reparative processes underlain by an unconscious feeling of guilt, which are therefore reorganising and creative for the intersubjective relationship and for the conjugal group.

Among the main potentially critical conjugal stages, I have identified: the living together or moving in together of the two conjugal partners in a common and shared space as an imaginary common body and psychic envelope requiring the inevitable setting into place of an organisation of domestic life and its vicissitudes; the institutionalisation of the couple through marriage; the formulation of the desire to, and the implementation of plans to, have a child, or its failure for various different reasons, such as sterility, even the lack of desire of one of the two; the birth of a child, or of the first child, therefore, the transition of the couple to the family and the virtually conflictual differentiation between conjugal or love couple and parental couple. To be mentioned also are some stages of the family life cycle, such as: the children's adolescence, inducing a *new experience* of the parents' oedipal conflict; the departure, then marriage of the children; the couple then once again find themselves living on a one-to-one basis; the aging of each one, with the cessation of professional activity of one partner, then both partners, determining the loss of a major object of investment, the work-object, having multiple implications for the psychic dynamic and economy of the retiree and of their couple; the birth of grandchildren and the new status of grandparent; finally the death of one of the partners.

About some evolving perspectives

Let us now discuss some evolving perspectives and essential conditions of the durability of a couple.

Wearing out and boredom within the couple

Parat (1967)[7] discusses a possible *wearing out* over time of the conjugal organisation, of oedipal structuration, that will be able to evolve into a relationship between the two partners reduced to a series of habits satisfying from the drive perspective, but that in the end locks them into an increasingly deadly, fixed, static, narrow world contrary to the preservation of a relationship involving a vigorous conjugal fantasy life and creativity.

Lemaire (1979) thinks that couples who accept and tolerate their wearing out do not "last". "They make relative living together possible, but they die as couples, even if they retain their legal façade, while on the contrary those that live are those who constantly restructure their bonds by abandoning their past with its outdated structure".[8]

Likewise, the couple can evolve towards a progressive de-erotisation between the two partners or towards the loss of certain qualities of one of the partners – whether it is a matter of an object of a genital relationship, of an object of tenderness, of a narcissistic or erotic object – something that inevitably perturbs the conjugal organisation.

Parat[9] furthermore invites us to observe that a possible disinvestment of the "world of others" can lead to locking the couple into a binary system, which, when it exceeds certain limits, ceases to belong to the oedipal organisation to regress towards a pregenital organisation underlain by a fixation. It regains the ambivalence and the aggression reintroduced into the couple in that manner, potentially containing the destruction of the love relationship.

For my part, *I will rather speak of the boredom that sets in over time, attesting to failure of their couple work.* It is of course a matter for couples that last, but at the cost of partial psychic death.

Why does one become bored in one's life as a couple? Is an element of boredom inevitable because it is intrinsic to conjugal temporality?

What does being bored in one's life as a couple signify on the metapsychological plane? What are the economic, dynamic and topic aspects of this?

Is it a matter of boredom on the individual-intrapsychic level experienced by one or both partners for different reasons, or within the intersubjective relation and/or within the conjugal group?

The depressive dimension of boredom in fact takes hold in the couple upon the instigation of one or both partners, and the balance of the economy of the drive intertwining is then distinctly tipped in favour of the death drive or of Eros' anti-regressive function. Eros' objectalising function therefore proves to be deficient, with a loss of capacities of investment of new objects. Couple work is work whose objectalising function must remain living and efficient, creative and symbolising, *impelling* the couple to renew itself, to invest new objects that are common and shared – but also personal and differentiated – to dream, to make plans, therefore, to project into the future, unlike the de-objectalising function, which has become predominant and leads to fixation and to locking into the present time or to regression towards a past that repeats itself, marked by traumatic or, just the opposite, glorious and idealised events.

Boredom can also be characterised by a distinct imbalance between the primary and secondary processes within the couple in favour of the latter. The secondarisation of conjugal life characterised, in particular, by a mechanical repetition of daily activities and factual communication devoid of affects, as well as a paucity, even extinction, of all fantasy life, also attests to the work of the death drive. Fantasy life can in fact die out in one or both partners, in the same way as the quest and desire for innovation and, therefore, the capacity to invest new objects can. There the partners' orality comes into play, manifesting itself through dissatisfaction, a need to change objects, for newness, to the detriment of anality, that fixes and immobilises and establishes itself in the long term and continuity.

Traumatisms, psychic disorganisations and somatisations happening within the couple

One cannot talk about conjugal life over the course of time without considering the possibility of psychic disorganisation or somatisation in one or both partners, fostered either by an event external to the couple, or by an event internal to one of them and/or by the difficulties and sufferings of conjugal life in its critical and very conflictual moments or their afterwardness.

Let us especially look at the somatisations. P. Marty (1990) brings up the movements of swinging between the two orders, psychic and somatic, of the psychosomatic unity of the human being and considers that the traumatisms are defined by "the quantity of disorganization that they produce and not by the quality of the event or of the situation producing them. A traumatism thus flows out of the relationship between excitation and the psychosomatic defense of the individual in question".[10]

He looks at two major processes of somatisation which create conditions of the development of somatic illnesses: somatic regression and progressive disorganisation both contribute to somatisations differing in nature and seriousness.

Both situate themselves within each partner's psychosomatic economy and within that of the couple. Numerous questions arise, which I shall not answer. For example: Do the partners represent for each other good protective shield objects or fantasy bearers able to make up for the deficiencies of the fantasising and representative activity of the other partner? Each one could thus represent for the other, or for the couple itself, good protection against any development of somatisation.

On the other hand, could the partner or the couple represent a source of excitation and of traumatisms of diverse kinds in certain critical and conflictual situations or periods? Could they therefore foster processes of somatisation in the partner? Would this be interpretable as symptomatic of a failure of couple work?

These are just examples of so many questions that could constitute the beginnings of research into a psychosomatics of a couple that would deserve to be undertaken.

Now, what about psychically living couples that last? Apart from the psychic economy and dynamic proper to each conjugal partner, essential factors of durability are to be taken into consideration.

Some factors of durability of a psychically living couple

The possibility of recurrently reliving the alternation of honeymoon phenomena followed by crisis

Indeed, Lemaire (1979)[11] stressed this alternation of honeymoon phenomena followed by crises, in an entangled and minor mode, marked in each partner by idealising splittings and mourning work, while Parat (1967) brought up "the possibility of reliving at variable intervals what deserves to be called a 'love state' perhaps in accordance with the 'narcissistic recharge' they involve".[12]

The erotic element and the narcissistic element

The pregenital component of the heterosexual relation of oedipal organisation involves an *erotic element* and a *narcissistic element*. Parat considered that this pregenital component of the conjugal and love investment is that which, like the tender investment, probably constitutes the least interchangeable, most specific element of the relationship, that which sometimes contributes most greatly to the constitution and consolidation of the love couple.

The erotic element seeks to regain and to realise old fantasies and pleasures, the partner being able to be used for this purpose as an object as oral as it is anal or phallic.

While the *narcissistic element* realises an overinvestment of the love-object corresponding to a displacement of the narcissism itself, this love-object then finds itself mixed up with the subject's internal objects, parental objects especially, that are then projected onto the chosen object. In its reciprocity, this overinvestment of the love-object is experienced as a personal narcissistic gain, the esteem received from the other person reinforcing one's self-esteem, which enables one to love oneself through identification with the other person who loves you.

The tender investment

This tender component proceeds from aim-inhibited erotic drives that must above all be characterised by their connection to the object. This restraining of the drive by itself would consist, according to A. Green[13] (1997), of an intrinsic modification of the erotic drives by the work of forces of separation, that is to say, by the work of the death drive, something that creates *ongoing and durable objectal investments*.

Naturally, but one cannot speak of this tender investment circulating between the two conjugal partners without referring to its beneficial regressive dimension, that is to say to the maternal tenderness. Indeed, P. C. Racamier (1969)[14] considered this maternal tenderness as a sensualised and successful derivative, on the one hand, of the primary narcissistic seduction occurring between the mother and her child, and, on the other hand, as the primary maternal preoccupation, the speciality of which is the envelope, something that justifies the role of this factor in the durability of the conjugal investment.

The current of aim-inhibited homosexual investment

M. Fain[15] (1967) held that life as a couple can enable the integration of the partners' homosexual libido. Moreover, he maintained that the most important fact is not satisfaction, but integration, that is to say "the feeling of being apt to be satisfied". In addition, this bond, which is both narcissistic and non-desexualised represents one of the rare elements durably conditioning a couple's union. However, the considerable force of the current of aim-inhibited homosexual investment within the couple can also be expressed through the tender and little erotised attachment of the two partners that will be accompanied by a significant limitation of their erotic life that becomes somewhat secondary and will contribute to the durability of the conjugal relationship.

The role of conjugal masochism or the sharing of the erogenous masochistic core of the two partners' Ego

Masochism enables one to bear, remember, relative non-satisfaction, immediate non-discharge (inherent in a durable object relationship). It is more specifically the Ego's masochistic core or primary erogenous masochism that makes possible the investment (the binding) of the excitation by making it acceptable. Thus, the continuity of the primary masochistic core in the Ego guarantees the psychic temporality-continuity by assuring the continuum of the excitation. Consequently, the assessment of the role and influence of the primary erogenous masochistic core at the heart of the object relationship proves essential, in particular, in order to think about the conditions of its durability, and more particularly that of every couple.

Indeed, to stay together over time, the two partners must tolerate conflicts, inevitable critical episodes, dissatisfactions, frustrations and disappointments of all kinds, as well as certain narcissistic wounds, to accept waiting and to defer satisfactions without considering an impulsive break-up. This is one of the major roles of the conjugal masochism proceeding from the sharing of the erogenous masochistic core of the partners' Ego that notably contributes to sustaining conjugal life.

Anality work of the two partners' Ego

Anality introduces time and continuity into the object relationship. It participates in the selection of the love-object, as well as in its fixation and in maintaining its tender and erotic investment, unlike orality. In addition, the Ego's anality work will synergically use the resources of its erogenous masochistic core to make the conjugal organisation last.

The role of seduction and of fantasising life

Maintaining diverse forms of mutual seduction contributes to nurturing desire and to stimulating fantasising activity, therefore, to keeping the couple psychically alive. While monogamy is associated with the partner's love investment, polygamous tendencies, which are more pronounced in men than in women (Parat),[16] die out, at least temporarily, when this investment is intense, owing to the overinvestment of the object. However, during the times when the relationship is less alive, this polygamous tendency can manifest itself in a fantasy mode and contribute to keeping the conjugal relationship alive, each partner identifying with the other in their free fantasy.

Moreover, the conjugal group must be able to assure fantasising production and circulation that will, in particular, stimulate the elaboration and realisation of common and shared projects.

"Dreaming", "creating", "building" together also contribute to preserving conjugal vitality, expressing the triumph of Eros and its objectalising function over the de-objectalising function of the death drive.

Maintaining the investment of the "world of others" outside the couple

The investment of the cultural and social environment through its diverse objects – be it of professional activity, the competitive and antagonistic value of which I have already underscored with the couple and the love-object, of children, of friends or of leisure activities – are going to play an equilibrating libidinal role and will be a source of drive vitality for conjugal life, capable of protecting it from the deadly dangers of boredom. Indeed, this complex and dynamic relationship with this other world of objects preserves the living and mobile homosexual identifications and exchanges, maintains the possibility of sublimated investments and correlative satisfactions. On the economic plane, the distribution of libidinal charges among these diverse objects will differ in quantity and quality and vary in terms of the periods in question.

However, this fluctuating investment can also sometimes be found at the origin of breakdowns of the couple's economic and dynamic equilibrium.

The possibility of breaking up

The worsening, on the one hand, of mutual aggressiveness without any possibility of orientation towards the "world of others" in a sublimated form and, on the other hand, the disinvestment of the partner gradually or suddenly leads to the separation of the two partners, therefore, to the break-up of their couple, which attests to the triumph of the death drive, whence it becomes necessary to bring up questions regarding the determining factors of this break-up.

Elaboration of a questioning process and reflection on separation and breaking up

From a psychoanalytic perspective, it is imperative to ask some preliminary fundamental questions:

- What do the desire to "separate" and then "separating" signify for conjugal partners?
- From whom, from what and why does one actually separate?
- From the partner, from the couple, from the love-object and from the couple-object?

One should differentiate between two types of objects of separation: that of the love-object and that of the couple-object.

The couple work required of each partner is committed to keeping the couple alive, which presumes, on the one hand, its durability and, on the other hand, its fantasy, affective and psychic vitality, therefore, the pre-eminence of Eros. On the other hand, its progressive dying out and/or its break-up would attest to a failure of couple work and to the triumph of the death drive. The economy of the drive intertwining proves central.

Let us look at the separation from the partner leading to conjugal break-up. The couple and couple work will be objectalised by the two partners' Eros.

On the other hand, through unbinding and disinvestment, the de-objectalis-ing function of the death drive will contribute to attacking each partner's couple work, leading to its failure if the quantitative relationship is in its favour, something that will manifest itself in multiple forms of suffering, even in a separation of the two partners and the subsequent conjugal break-up.

Separation from the conjugal partner or love-object

Who precisely is this love-object? Whom does he or she represent in the subject's fantasised internal world?

Remember that *the love-object* is characterised by its historicity and the work of its specific choice in reference to one or some fantasy objects of pregenital origin, the primary maternal object, but also of oedipal origin, the maternal and paternal objects.

So, we could relate the choice of love-object and its psychic determi-nants to the desire to separate from it.

Why separate from it?

We already know that the love-object must satisfy a certain number of needs, desires and expectations of a narcissistic, pregenital and genital kind and help the subject's Ego reinforce its defensive system. Inasmuch as it is an internal object, it must of course carry out certain functions within the subject's Ego. Does it always fulfil them?

Some questions then arise: that of the economic relationships between satisfactions and frustrations, tensions of displeasure, even sufferings, but also that of the mobility of each of the partners' libidinal economy – between homosexual and heterosexual, objectal and narcissistic invest-ments; as well as that of the economy of the drive intertwining between Eros and the death drive.

In short, does the subject always find more benefits there than dis-satisfactions with their partner or not?

Furthermore, has that love-object already totally or partially satisfied the desires and expectations? If the answer is affirmative, how is one to understand an evolution towards dissatisfactions? Would it be a matter of a personal evolution on each one's part involving changes, as much in their needs and expectations, therefore, in their psychic economy, as in the responses provided by the partner?

Each one's psychic evolution is inevitably going to contribute to desta-bilising the couple's dynamic and economic balance, by its personal crises and the reactivation of conflicts, in particular.

Break-up of the couple and separation from its intrapsychic representative, the internal couple-object

Remember, the couple-object becomes a new internal object establishing relationships of conflictuality with, on the one hand, the external object, the conjugal reality, and, on the other hand, with the infantile mnesic representation of the real parental couple and the idealised couple-object. Relationships of qualitative comparison and evaluation will be at work and generate tensions within each partner's Ego and between the two partners.

On the groupal level, the separation of the two partners leading to the couple's break-up represents the breaking of the *conjugal narcissistic contract*. The couple's narcissistic foundations are therefore called into question and the fundamental conflict between each partner's narcissistic requirements and those of the couple returns.

Did this contract become a destructive narcissistic pact for one of the partners whose psychic economy evolved to the point of having to separate – just as a breakdown of offensive and defensive alliances also takes place?

Have defensive alliances become useless or pathogenic, perverse or alienating, for one or both partners?

What roles could the representations of each of the partners' parental couple play?

When a partner breaks up their couple, is it exclusively a matter of their own couple, or would there not be also an act of fantasised break-up of the intrapsychic parental couple underlain by an unconscious infantile fantasy of separating the parents, therefore of attacking, of destroying, their erotic couple in connection with a primal scene that is unbearable because the level of excitation is too intense, even sadistic, but also because it acts to exclude in connection with oedipal failure and its correlative narcissistic wounds?

This fantasy can be living in each one of us and, once acted upon, it is accompanied both by an unconscious satisfaction signifying revenge and reparative triumph on the narcissistic plane, as well as by an unconscious feeling of guilt.

Consequently, forming a couple in order to break it up later is perhaps also destroying the internal parental couple experienced as a persecuting internal object that must be annihilated.

Just as an individual chooses their conjugal partner and they construct their couple with their own parental representations charged with affects by favouring certain of them, the individual also separates "from them", or separates from certain of them, to choose others during the possible construction of a new couple.

Thus, the relationship of each partner to their own parental representations will therefore contribute to the future of their couple.

Nevertheless, the two partners can meet around a common and shared fantasy to create a couple better than that of their parents, which then becomes an internal and external reality, but the former can then be a source of an unconscious feeling of guilt that will manifest itself in a need for punishment – expressing itself by a failure of couple work and then in a break-up that brings relief on the unconscious plane.

What about the love couple becoming a parental couple? The breaking up of a parental couple falls within the framework of the structural conflictuality between the couple and the family, thus determining the existence of "anti-family" couples and "anti-couple" families and therefore bearing destructive movements between these two antagonistic terms.

In this situation, family unity is threatened, its bonds will be destroyed and the children will suffer from it – and the parental couple will be responsible for this, which is all the more a cause of feelings of guilt for the parents since their parental couple took precedence over their love couple. This is why their failure is all the more violent.

In this painful and critical context, each partner identifies with their children and suffers for and with them, which then reactivates their wounds caused by the real or fantasised separation of their own parents.

One also realises that the ideal of a close family is much more invested than that of a love couple. Why? It is the oedipal child in us who would feel guilty giving priority to investing in its love couple, due to its historically transgressive meaning, rather than prioritising its parental role and the family, therefore, the children.

Another question to consider is that concerning a gender gap between men and women confronted with the actual separation of the partners and also conjugal break-up. This question can arise, for example, in terms of level and of quality of investment in each one's couple work and, more generally, in terms of drive economy and differentiated distribution of the objects of investment in each partner, among the Ego, the love-object, the couple-object and the objects belonging to the "world of others", notably, the work-object, children, friends and leisure activities, in particular.

What about the suffering inherent in the separation and conjugal break-up?

It is certainly composite and does not exclude an unconscious satisfaction when it is correlative to an unconscious fantasised attack of the intrapsychic parental couple as we have envisaged it.

For a better understanding, it would be appropriate to distinguish between the suffering inherent in the separation from the love-object and that connected with conjugal break-up.

Indeed, the love-object is invested in a fundamentally ambivalent fashion, while the couple-object will above all receive a sublimated homosexual and narcissistic investment from both partners.

So, during a separation, participating in a movement of drive disunion between Eros and the destruction drives, the hostile component of ambivalence with regard to the love-object frees itself fully. In addition, there is a worsening of certain structural conflictualities, essential dynamic components of the intersubjective relationship, while what has been repressed and split returns to consciousness. There are modes of object relation, such as that of an anal-sadistic nature, which predominate and the psychotic virtualities of the relationship, notably of a paranoid type, externalise, determining violent and major projective movements, the love-object subsequently becoming both an internal and external persecutor threatening the Ego's dynamic and economy. Likewise, an experience of destruction of the internal world and of narcissistic failure manifests itself in each one. All of that contributes to the suffering, but also to a certain extent proves to be necessary in order to accomplish the operation of separation. *Every separation in fact requires the mobilisation of each partner's destructive drive motions in order to break these intersubjective bonds.*

On the other hand, conjugal break-up with the correlative loss of the couple-object is much more painful because of its major narcissistic investment. "In it one loses a good part of oneself", which has then become bad and threatening, but which remains partially idealised, and the mourning work will be all the more difficult and painful for that. The function of the conjugal Ideal is also attacked and the return of what has been repressed and what has been split/denied can cause considerable damage.

I will close this question-asking process with one last question to which I will propose the beginnings of a response.

Separation work

From an economic perspective, it is a matter of a traumatic situation of loss of both the love-object and the couple-object.

This mourning work will thus have to consist of accepting the painful reality of separation and break-up, therefore, of this double loss – as much of "this" chosen love-object as of "this" couple-object – experienced as a form of destruction as personal (both narcissistic and objectal) as it is groupal-conjugal. This will necessarily involve a drive disinvestment-detachment mobilising destructive drive motions that, on the one hand, will enable each of the separated partners to realise a narcissistic reinvestment of their Ego – thus contributing to the restoration of a much more satisfying economy and dynamic as well as to a reconstruction of their world of internal objects – and, on the other hand, to be able to invest "new objects" libidinally, such as a new love-object. Finally, if the couple is parental, this work must be able to pacify the relationship so as to make it liveable, something that serves to comfort their children, but also makes for exchanges between "good parents" that are less ambivalent and are freed from narcissistic issues.

Let us note that this work can be based on a relatively good investment of objects of the "world of others", protecting from depressive dangers, such as the work-object and its environment, the children, the circle of close friends and leisure activities, for example.

However, separation from one's partner and conjugal break-up may be distinctly beneficial, even life-saving, often attesting to psychic progress in one of the partners, after a considerable effort finally enabling them to be free of perverse or alienating defensive alliances. This suffering partner then makes genuine maturational progress by winning their autonomy. Often, this separation proves possible thanks to individual analytic work.

I will stop here and turn to the second part of my study, work with couples.

Notes

1 É. Smadja, *Le couple et son histoire* (Presses universitaires de France, 2011, in French); as *The Couple: A Pluridisciplinary Story* (Routledge, 2016, in English).
2 C. Parat, "L'organisation œdipienne du stade genital", *Revue française de psychanalyse*, 31, 5–6 (1967).
3 C. Parat, "L'organisation œdipienne du stade genital", *Revue française de psychanalyse*, 31, 5–6 (1967), p. 794.
4 J.-G. Lemaire, *Le couple, sa vie, sa mort* (Payot, 1979).
5 B. Rosenberg, *Masochisme gardien de la vie, masochisme mortifère* (Presses universitaires de France, 1991).
6 A. Ruffiot, "Le couple and l'amour. De l'originaire au groupal", in A. Eiguer (ed.), *La thérapie psychanalytique du couple* (Bordas, 1984).
7 C. Parat, "L'organisation œdipienne du stade genital", *Revue française de psychanalyse*, 31, 5–6 (1967).
8 J.-G. Lemaire, *Le couple, sa vie, sa mort* (Payot, 1979), p. 337.
9 C. Parat, "L'organisation œdipienne du stade genital", *Revue française de psychanalyse*, 31, 5–6 (1967).
10 P. Marty, *La psychosomatique de l'adulte* (Presses universitaires de France, 1990), p. 79.
11 J.-G. Lemaire, *Le couple, sa vie, sa mort* (Payot, 1979).
12 C. Parat, "L'organisation œdipienne du stade genital", *Revue française de psychanalyse*, 31, 5–6 (1967), p. 805.
13 A. Green, *The Chains of Eros, The Sexual in Psychoanalysis* (Karnac, 2008, in English); translation of *Les chaînes d'Eros, l'actualité du sexuel* (Odile Jacob, 1997).
14 P. C. Racamier, *L'inceste et l'incestuel* (Les éditions du Collège, 1995).
15 M. Fain, "Intervention sur le rapport de C. Parat", Revue française de psychanalyse, 31, 5–6 (1967), 822.
16 C. Parat, "L'organisation œdipienne du stade genital", *Revue française de psychanalyse*, 31, 5–6 (1967).

Part II
Work with couples

Introduction to Part II

Psychoanalytic work with couples is an example of *transposition* (J. L. Donnet, 2005)[1] of *transference* (R. Roussillon, 2008),[2] one of the fields of "applied psychoanalysis" receiving the general method issuing from the individual cure (D. Anzieu, 1975; R. Kaës, 2015).[3]

This *transference* will thus produce the setting up of an analysing arrangement, of an "analytic site" (Donnet) for the couple that will become a "specific analytic object". But this *transference*, as Roussillon suggests to us, is also that of a principle of listening: we will be attentive both to each partner's free association, which will reveal their intrapsychic bonds to us, and to the free association circulating between the two partners, revealing to us both the groupal and intersubjective dimension of their bonds.

Moreover, this groupal analytic situation in which the members can see themselves and see the analyst induces a specific type of regression and particularities of the transferential process resulting in some specific characteristics of the modes of listening, of intervention and of interpretation.

Consequently, being a psychoanalyst with a couple will present similarities and differences with a patient in a typical cure, or closer at hand, with a patient face to face as well as with a group. Anzieu[4] (1975) laid down three sorts of rules guiding his psychoanalytic manner of proceeding with groups:

- those forming the basis of a psychoanalytic thought procedure;
- those enabling the inauguration of a psychoanalytic process;
- those governing the psychoanalytic interpretation in this situation.

We can also draw inspiration from these rules to establish the bases of our psychoanalytic work with couples. Thus, in a situation with a couple established in accordance with a psychoanalytic model by a psychoanalyst having a psychoanalytic thought procedure, a work of a psychoanalytic nature can from then on be performed with the patients as well as with the analyst.

DOI: 10.4324/9781003635093-10

The basis of our psychoanalytic thought procedure, in fact, consists of our envisaging conscious and unconscious conjugal psychic reality as being constituted of three connected and interdependent structuro-functional levels: intrapsychic-individual, intersubjective and groupal, each one involving its organisers, its formations, its dynamic conflictualities and its economic aspects.

The rules enabling the inauguration of a psychoanalytic process are the two fundamental rules of non-omission or free association and of abstinence which must be adjusted in terms of the particular characteristics that the couples represent.

Finally, some principles will guide the psychoanalytic interpretation in this specific situation with couples. In our opinion, this groupal analytic situation is going to determine certain characteristics of the transference, which differ from those of the individual arrangement that will lead to a specific kind of interpretative work:

- The first is an individual transference of each partner onto the analyst.
- The second is an intertransference or lateral transference of the two partners between themselves that is constitutive of an intertransferential neurosis.
- Third is that of the transference of the couple, as a group, onto the analyst.
- Finally, a transference of each partner and of the couple onto the *therapeutic group* formed by the two partners, the couple *and* the analyst. This new "object" that the therapeutic group constitutes will be invested as a fantasised and libidinal object by each person and by the couple and it will be one of the objects of the countertransference of the analyst.

Much later, Kaës (2015)[5] would also characterise the group psychoanalytic arrangement and the work it makes possible. This will help us to reflect even better on the principles and modalities of our work.

> The theory of the three spaces of psychic reality and the model of the groupal psychic apparatus form the metapsychological and methodological framework of a complex conception of transference, of the associative processes, of the listening and of the interpretation in the groups.
> The transferential configurations in the group situation, the correlations among the objects of transference, the particularities of the associative process and of the interdiscursivity determine a process of *psychic work* having specific modalities and results.[6]

We will return to this later on in Part II, Chapter 3, which is specifically devoted to the modalities of our work with couples.

Before this, we will present the diverse circumstances of consultation, in Part II, Chapter 1, the opening chapter for this Part, followed by, in Part II, Chapter 2, the characteristics of the preliminary interviews, from the first contact made, up until the presentation of the analytic framework to the consulting couple.

Notes

1 J. L Donnet, *La situation analysante* (Presses universitaires de France, 2005).
2 R. Roussillon, *Le jeu et l'entre-je(u)* (Presses universitaires de France, 2008).
3 D. Anzieu, *Le groupe et l'inconscient* (Dunod, 1984; first published 1975); translated as *The Group and the Unconscious* (Routledge, 2014).
4 R. Kaës, *L'extension de la psychanalyse* (Dunod, 2015).
5 R. Kaës, *L'extension de la psychanalyse* (Dunod, 2015).
6 R. Kaës, *L'extension de la psychanalyse* (Dunod, 2015), p. 185.

1 Suffering couples and the circumstances of consultation

Through information disseminated by the media about the existence of various kinds of conjugal help (conjugal advice, therapies, medical consultation, sexology advice, advice from "shrinks"), couples are seeking professional help at an increasingly young age and increasingly early in their life together as a couple, most often upon the woman's initiative. Multiple causes of dissatisfaction, critical personal and conjugal phases, and conflictualities exacerbated by those critical periods and events are the principal motives for this. More specifically, let us consider the following situations.

The relationship between the two partners is experienced as inadequate, difficult, complicated, blocked and they suffer from this

The two partners say that they do not, or no longer, understand each other. The minute they open their mouths, they end up in a violent fight. Would this be a "symptomatic" way of creating a necessary distance between them so that, thanks to this inadequacy, they are protected in this way against dreaded latent symbiotico-fusional aspirations (J.-G. Lemaire)?[1] Indeed, not communicating, not understanding each other, arguing are, in fact, also ways of limiting the potentially dangerous, depersonalising density of the relationship.

Martine, 35 years old and Louis, 40 years old, came to consult me regarding Louis's angry outbursts, which troubled their life as a couple considerably, becoming an object of conjugal conflict and revelatory of latent conflicts that we were going to discover together.

They have been together for ten years. However, they lived together for eight years and have been married for two years.

Both work a great deal and fail to take very much advantage of their free time. Martine in fact complains that Louis comes home late every evening, that they do not enjoy themselves and rarely go out together, and above all that he is reserved, not talking enough about how his day went,

DOI: 10.4324/9781003635093-11

about his work, about his feelings, quite simply about himself. Actually, she complains about their verbal and affective exchanges, which she finds so poor and unsatisfactory.

Louis explains that after a long day at work he needs a time of silence to take some necessary distance from both his excessively mentally demanding work and his wife. It is a time of mental restoration. Moreover, he thinks that work should not enter into his private space. There are different spaces and times to differentiate, to separate, without allowing contamination. He feels his wife's questions are intrusive and her requests invasive. This is why he must protect himself from these dangers by creating some distance, mainly achieved by his silence.

I would find that his wife's demands conjure up for him those of his mother, often issued as directives in an authoritarian manner. In this way, his wife would therefore represent a dangerous mother figure from whom he must protect himself. Martine does not understand Louis's need for silence, which she experiences and interprets as a form of rejection, a lack of interest in her, abandonment, reactivating the disinvestment and traumatic abandonment that her father inflicted upon her when she was a child, and that her mother, with whom "little Martine" identifies in this painful situation, also experienced. Moreover, with Louis, she re-enacts her need to establish a symbiotico-fusional relationship with her mother.

Finally, I understand that Louis's angry outbursts express his inability to tell Martine, out of fear of hurting her, of his temporary need to remain a little alone in her presence by means of his protective, restorative silence, but also of the pressure of his fantasised expectations that weigh on him. He is in fact afraid that she will interpret this as a kind of abandonment, indifference and that she will then react aggressively. So, he restrains himself, holds back, then, after a while, when some insignificant situation arises, he explodes.

My work to reformulate, to verbalise these affects, these fantasies and these interpretations enables me to clarify and correct their pathogenic mutual projections. It also helped them to reduce considerably the frequency and intensity of these outbursts, making them pointless from then on. This opened the way to the verbalisation of latent conflicts and things left unsaid, protected and kept at a distance by the manifest symptom of "Louis's angry outbursts".

As concerns erotic life

It may be a matter of loss of desire and of any form of seduction, but also of certain forms of suffering (frigidity or painful intercourse in the case of women, impotency and premature ejaculation in the case of men), often presented as being the case with one of partners. They may also represent another form of limitation against the density of the relationship and its fusional risks experienced in satisfactory sexual union.

Beatrice, 40 years old and Marc, 43 years old. We already presented Beatrice and Marc in Part I, Chapter 4, which was devoted to the groupal level to illustrate conjugal compromise formations and the phoric function.

An ongoing or too recurrent conflictual form of communication

While this mode of conflictual relationship can be understood as a symptom, the making of a compromise, a mutual reaction of identity and narcissistic affirmation, reinforcing thus the insufficient, therefore threatened, psychic individual boundaries by each partner (Lemaire),[2] I see it as "noisily" expressing the fundamental antagonisms between Ego/love-object, identity/alterity, narcissism/objectality, and that of the difference of the sexes, in particular.

Thomas, 32 years old and Claire, 25 years old had separated temporarily in order to think things over before coming to consult me.

There are too many conflicts between them, too many complaints and reproaches, actually too many misunderstandings.

> "Thomas", Claire says, "is too passive at home, never decides any-
> thing, doesn't get involved in anything. He's a couch potato slumped
> on the sofa watching the TV. He is tyrannical, makes me wear the
> clothes he likes, rather sexy ones, to go out, without taking my clothes
> into account".

In addition, Claire complains about organising all their home life, therefore about Thomas's passivity and would like him to take the initiative from time to time. Likewise, she also complains about his lack of verbal exchanges, about having to make conversation. He behaves like a child with her, while she needs a man to rely on. He readily admits this, but cannot do much about it.

Last year, they decided to try to save their life together as a couple, which was then mired in a state of ongoing crisis. That did not change anything. In fact, it was their respective parents who took charge of and organised their marriage, making them feel that "their" marriage had been taken away from them. In addition, it was also the parents, Claire's parents, who bought her an apartment in which they both live and which Claire decorated in accordance with her taste. Moreover, he does not really feel at home.

They met at a party among friends. He was a 26-year-old engineer at the time and Claire, barely 19 years old, was only in her first year of design school. She had been immediately seduced by the image he represented for her, what he personified for her, the "prince charming" she was waiting for. It was love at first sight for both of them. He said that at the beginning of their life together Claire's admiration for him made him omnipotent, invincible, indomitable, while Claire very quickly felt the desire to devote her life to him. They moved in together shortly afterwards, thanks to the purchase of an apartment by the father of Claire (who was living in a one-room apartment). The routineness of daily life, bearable in the beginning, quickly became invasive. Then, Thomas encountered some professional difficulties that made him doubt his self-worth, his competency. He could not talk to Claire about it, who had to preserve a beautiful image of him as a strong man exclusively anchored in success. He was then seduced by a young enterprising woman whom he knew through his work and increasingly "amorous" exchanges ensued, which Claire discovered by chance. This was traumatic for her and for their life as a couple. Something was definitively *broken*: Claire's absolute trust in Thomas and Thomas's feeling of omnipotence.

From then on, Claire no longer trusted him and Thomas could not rid himself of feelings of guilt, which grew unbearable over the years. In fact, he saw himself as being a "bad boy" who had never satisfied his parents' expectations and demands, except when it came to success at school. Thomas was the youngest sibling and he rebelled against his parents very early, unlike his older siblings. So this "bad boy" had always lived with this unconscious belief. From this point of view, meeting Claire was "therapeutic", because he no longer experienced himself as "bad" but, suddenly, became "good". However, this tenacious belief was going to re-emerge during this episode of extraconjugal seduction.

Thus, Claire's reproaches were reactivating this image of the "bad boy" who did not do what was expected of him. As for Claire, Thomas's passivity and his lack of investment in their conjugal life, with her, even though he loves her deeply, moreover, was reactivating the abandonment Claire had felt by her father because of his multiple professional trips, which were traumatic for her. She had found herself locked up alone with her mother for weeks on end, locked into a dual alienating relationship, stifled by her mother's demands, her desubjectivating, lethal entreaties. This is why, in the presence of Thomas, she was reliving in another way the traumatic abandonment her father had recurrently inflicted upon her during the first ten years of her life. While they had thought and hoped at the very beginning of their conjugal relationship to be able to "treat" and "repair" their early wounds together with the other person and within their relationship, they only ended up reactivating them. This was in fact a failure of their *couple work*.

In addition, these multiple complaints and reproaches caused conflicts that were only exacerbations of some of their structural conflictualities within the framework of intertransferential movements: in particular between identity/alterity, narcissism/objectality and masculine/feminine.

Identity/alterity: There was no genuine psychic recognition of the other person's alterity, of their differences with respect to themselves, despite intellectual   recognition   through   speech.   The   uniqueness   and

distinctiveness, as well as the difficulties, of the other person were therefore not accepted.

Narcissism/objectality: There was a conflict between individual interests
and the interests of the other person and of the couple. Claire had "for-
gotten herself" in her hyper-investment of Thomas and of her life with
him as a couple and she suffered from that because, in return, she did not
reap narcissistic benefits from her husband while he was focused on himself and on his narcissistic fragility that Claire and her role in the couple
needed to help him repair.

Masculine/feminine: If Thomas must play a masculine protective and
seductive role with Claire, she above all represents for him a "feminine
narcissistic double", which she must remain – as he himself wishes. This is
a way of satisfying, on the level of fantasy, his feminine desires by identifying with her by way of projective identification. But this is also a
modality of narcissistic reparation, of being proud of having, of being with
and of showing his friends and others his so seductive and charming wife.
The phallic stakes are "sizeable". For Claire, her feminine desires of
seduction, of active passivity and of "letting herself be led" by *her* man,
virile, enterprising and reassuring, were not being satisfied. Nonetheless,
by identifying with her father, as well as her mother, although in a different way, she was satisfying her masculine desires with Thomas,
although they conflicted with her feminine desires, something that was
exacerbating and contributing to the outbreak of conjugal conflicts.

Finally, since their life as a couple was growing worse, and both of them
were considering themselves incapable of finding a satisfactory solution,
Thomas suddenly decided, from one day to the next, to leave their apartment, leaving Claire a letter explaining his departure.

A conflictual relationship in a male couple

John, 32 years old and Mark, 40 years old, consulted me because for several
months they had been having unbearable conflicts threatening them with
a new break-up, which they did not want. They had lived together as a
couple for three years and had already contended with two brief episodes
of separation, each time upon Mark's initiative. They do not frequent the
Parisian gay milieu, which they reject, in part owing to their shared,
common conception of fidelity and conjugal exclusivity, as distinguished,
notably, from having possible multiple partners.

John felt neglected by Mark and reproached him for not investing
enough in their life as a couple. Thus, he considered that Mark was above
all wrapped up in his work, leaving very early and returning fairly late
every day of the week, while during the weekend, he "just vegetated",
hanging around in the apartment, expressing reticence about going out to
go to the cinema, to an exhibition, or to eat out with friends. So, John had
been feeling more and more alone, obliged then to do the main part of the

housework and suffering emotionally from lack of attention and affection from Mark. Their sex life was going downhill. Moreover, John often expressed feelings of jealousy with respect to the special, "very affectionate" relationships that Mark maintained with co-workers, both men and women, which John considered as being to his detriment, all the more so because Mark was being less and less loving towards him. This was why he was more frequently acting possessively, which Mark felt was invasive and stifling.

For his part, Mark complained about feeling gradually locked up in his conjugal relationship and too controlled, kept under surveillance by John, whose growing jealousy was keeping him from seeing his friends as he pleased. He felt he had to account for himself every time he dared to go out alone, without him, and every evening he felt apprehensive about returning home, fearing additional reproaches from his companion. That situation was becoming intolerable and was making him unhappy. He no longer felt he was his old self, he who was so jovial, talkative, surrounded by friends, taking part in festivities, reading extensively and with such passion. He had begun to feel anxious about having to tell John about late evening meetings or work weekends, which he felt obliged to cancel from time to time.

This was why Mark felt his partner was completely treating him as a child, embodying a parental figure, just as John felt himself to be a neglected wife abandoned by his companion. They had both found themselves at an impasse.

In the course of our work together, certain elements of Mark's and John's personal and family lives enabled us to uncover some intertransferential movements at work in the construction and functioning of their conjugal life, shedding light in particular on their diverse objects of suffering.

Thus, John had lived in a family of four brothers and sisters – he being the youngest – in which his mother had felt that her husband had completely lost interest in her, being principally caught up in his work and extraprofessional activities, composed of leisure activities, friendships and extraconjugal relationships. She had been completely responsible for managing the home and family life and had sought to compensate for the painful lack of love from her husband by seeking affection and gratitude from her children, unfortunately by being omnipresent, something they had felt was suffocating, even invasive and intrusive. This had above all been the case with the young John who had had to leave home at an early age to protect himself from it. In short, he had experienced both disinterestedness, equivalent to abandonment, on the part of his father and an invasive suffocation, threatening his subjectivation-individuation, on the part of his mother. Moreover, he had not been able to find any structuring support from his brothers and sisters, among whom a rather fierce rivalry had reigned, essentially concerning success at school, which was the only thing that aroused their father's interest.

John's leaving his family's home had been life saving, and he had been able to flourish as a student living in a different city.

The discovery of his attraction to young men had taken place during John's teen years and it had not been until after leaving home that he had been able to satisfy his desire to have romantic and sexual affairs with other men, something that had contributed to constructing his male identity, the process of which had for the most part been impeded within his family.

However, John's coming-out met with radical, massive rejection by his parents, as well as by both of his brothers, something that would distance him all the more from them.

After studying law very successfully, John had decided to become a legal consultant at a major bank for which he had been working up to that time.

John had undergone several experiences of conjugal life, but they had been quite unsatisfying, because his partners had had multiple partners, something that he had never tolerated, whence the frequent break-ups.

As for Mark, he had grown up with an older brother and both parents engrossed in their work. His mother had been practically non-existent, while his father, bad-tempered and unpredictable, had been much more present and had taken on some of the housework. So the two brothers had been left to their own devices at too early an age, their parents granting them freedom and many responsibilities. They never did anything really stupid though and had had to mature very quickly. Mark had been an excellent student and was accepted into one of the elite engineering schools. He is presently a technical director for a prestigious public works firm.

After having had some particularly disappointing sexual experiences with young women, starting at the age of 18, he became aware of his desires for men and had had frequent, brief affairs, they too just as unsatisfying, but for other reasons, notably affective. He had in fact discovered his immense emotional needs that these men could not help him satisfy. His coming-out had been unproblematic, and both his parents and his brother had accepted it showing a great deal of understanding.

He has often consulted community meeting sites on the web but, just like John, he does not frequent the gay milieux.

They had met one another a little more than three years earlier through an internet site and both of them had practically fallen "head over heels in love". They had experienced a "honeymoon" period, which had made them decide very quickly to live together, at first in John's apartment. Then they wanted to move into a new place, chosen, furnished and decorated together. They were often together, and their love life was fully satisfying to both of them. For a time, Mark disinvested his job, his friends, his reading, to devote himself to John and their life as a couple.

Then after a few months, Mark was overcome with feelings of invasion and suffocation, which caused him a considerable amount of anxiety. The distancing of himself from his friends and the relative disinvestment of his work aroused feelings of depression in him. While he had discovered and gained something new and important from the present romantic relationship, he suddenly became aware that he had lost something just as important and structuring for him: the investment in his job, his friends, major sources of support, and his leisure activities. His life with John then involved its share of alienation, desubjectivisation, even relative depersonalisation. "He felt less and less himself". He then began to grow apart from John and to reinvest in what was essential to himself, something that John experienced as estrangement, and then as abandonment, to which John reacted by reproaching Mark and adopting increasingly possessive and invasive attitudes, which would make Mark take refuge all the more in work and silence.

In the course of our work together, we discovered in particular that, through his possessive and invasive attitudes, John was identifying with his mother in the relationship she had maintained with him as a child and as an adolescent. But, by adopting these attitudes, he had also been seeking Mark's love, as someone representing a transferential father-figure who was not interested in him. The affective warmth and maternal care that John offered Mark enabled the latter to try to "repair" profound suffering from maternal deprivation. But it had become too much. Likewise, while John was identifying him with a distant father-figure who had rejected him, Mark himself was identifying with the mother of his childhood, all but absent from family and conjugal life. In his life with John, he had then been reliving this early traumatic experience, which had caused unhealed narcissistic wounds.

He could not satisfy John's excessive demands, which also found expression in their sex life.

John also complained about Mark's belittling and excluding him in various different ways, especially in the presence of friends and acquaintances. It was a matter of Mark's sense of humour, which John failed to understand. With respect to this, Mark became aware of his identification with his father, described as brusque, with distinctly sadistic tendencies, which could be disguised by humour. These painful situations reactivated John's feelings of being excluded by his father and the belittlement inflicted by his two older brothers. He was reliving feelings of injustice and incomprehension.

Some months of work at verbalising and achieving a flow of affects and phantasies brought about an awareness of several things and brought to light unconscious contents and processes present in each of them and within their life as a couple. However, Mark and John were also exposed to conjugal and individual resistances that they considered insurmountable, which proved determinant in their decision to break up definitively, "aware of what it was that had been going on", thus breaking off their joint therapy.

Crisis correlative to the transition from a conjugal couple to a parental couple, from the couple to the family

Lise, 40 years old and Sylvain, 38 years old, had been experiencing a serious crisis that began a few months after the birth of their first child, Pierre.

It had already been five years since they met. For several months they experienced a "honeymoon", which made them decide very quickly to live together in Lise's one-room apartment. She then expressed her desire for a child, sustained by the conviction that very early on she had seen in Sylvain the father she was dreaming for her children. Sylvain accepted, because it increased his sense of self-worth, but not without feeling some reticence, which he felt unable to express in the face of Lise's enthusiasm and out of his desire to make her happy.

Pierre was born one year after they met. This was a source of a total happiness, something unknown before then to Lise, who thus became a happy, fulfilled mother through this son.

Together they formed a new couple to the detriment of her conjugal couple with Sylvain, whom she asked to play his role as father so as to form a parental couple responding their son's every need. In so doing, she abandoned their life as a love couple and Sylvain felt deserted, which reactivated in him anxieties of abandonment and exclusion and a painful sibling rivalry with his younger brother, overinvested by his own parents.

The first symptom of this conjugal crisis linked to the transition from couple to family was Lise's loss of any erotic desire for Sylvain. From then on, she became a mother finding fulfilment in a symbiotico-fusional relation with her son. Her erotic investment in fact transformed and shifted from the couple to her motherhood and the relationship with her son. Sylvain's suffering was expressed in reproaches and growing hostility regarding aspects of their home life. While Lise reproached him for not participating sufficiently in their home life, going shopping, helping with the chores, which she had to do alone from that point on.

Faced with this disastrous situation, he decided to invest more and more in his professional activity and his leisure activities, some of which he no longer shared with Lise.

In fact, in Lise, this mode of investment of motherhood responded to a need to show her mother that she was no longer the irresponsible, imma-ture, capricious girl she had so often been said to be, but that she too was capable of fully being a woman, meaning first of all a mother, and, what is more, much better than her own mother. The oedipal issue was therefore primordial for Lise, while Sylvain was experiencing trauma for the second time, the first time having been inflicted by his own mother when she imposed a little brother upon him when he was only two years old. This trauma of the birth of his little brother would therefore be reactivated by the birth of his son accompanied by the hyper-investment of his wife to become an exclusive mother.

Behind the increase in self-worth attached to Sylvain's desire to become a father hid his latent desire to remain the preferred son of his mother and to form a lasting couple with her, at the risk of confronting the threat of castration.

Psychic and/or physical conjugal violence

Psychic and/or physical conjugal violence must raise questions for us about their intertransferential/transferential meaning and their dimension, as unconscious fantasied as it is of pure discharge of excitation devoid of representative content.

Corinne, 38 years old and Luke, 40 years old, had been living together for ten years. They were the parents of a 6-year-old child named Paul. They could no longer talk with each other without becoming aggressive and their exchanges were accompanied by violent reproaches and ongoing mutual denigration, which drained them to the point of contemplating separation, which, moreover, they could not carry out. On the other hand, there had never been any physical violence between them.

Our work over the course of the sessions enabled us to discover the intertransferential aspects of their conjugal violence and the unconscious representations underlying it inherent in their personal life stories.

Corinne had lived in a very rowdy "expanded" family with many people (uncles and aunts, cousins, friends) who came and went, little privacy, parents living together, but maintaining their independence. Her father treated her fairly tenderly – which she had been able to interpret as a form of seduction underlain by an unconscious incestuous fantasy – although he was also fairly firm and demanding, while her mother was particularly denigrating, even psychically abusive. And yet, this little girl admired her mother, invested with an omnipotence, but unfortunately haughty and too distant. How was she to find fulfilment as a woman with such a mother? Only somatic events made it possible for Corinne, at the risk of endangering herself, to capture her mother's attention and interest, finally devoting a little time to her daughter.

As for Luke, he grew up in a lethal family environment, marked by boredom, his parents' quasi-silence and rigorous discipline. Disinvested by her husband very early, Luke's mother was entirely invasively, even vampirically, devoted to her two children. His father organised the activities of family life in a very ritualised way, but took little interest in his wife and children. He is described as a hard, severe man, most often reproachful and deprecating towards his wife and children. At home, the children did not speak. Moreover, no one was interested in what they might feel or think. In addition, Luke described himself as being a phobic child with regard to the external world outside his family, not having friends.

Meeting Corinne was good for him, even "therapeutic", because she brought him the life he was missing so much, but with some excesses. In addition, she played a counterphobic role in relation to him, which he needed in order finally to confront the world and go out into it less dangerously. Through her, he was able to meet many people, because she loved to organise meals with friends, outings, trips, at the risk of invading him and draining him as well, something for which he reproached her.

By meeting Luke, Corinne was able to rein in some of her excessive liveliness, which expressed itself in a diffuse, draining hyperactivity sometimes putting her in danger, just as she found in him a protective, stable and reliable man. On the other hand, she found a maternal transferential figure again in his abusive, deprecating language and attitudes, all the more frequent since Luke felt estranged from Corinne, at the time very invested in her multiple activities and her telephone conversations with her friends, which he experienced as a form of maternal abandonment. He had not actually experienced that with his mother, who was entirely devoted to her two children. However, he needed Corinne's exclusive attention to continue to feel that he existed, but when Luke was verbally aggressive with Corinne, he was identifying with the father of his childhood and replaying the verbal violence that his father had inflicted upon him, which was traumatic for him at the time. In like manner, he experienced the many activities that Corinne organised with a feeling of being locked up and stifled. This was something that, moreover, he had already experienced as a child with his father, whence Corinne's finding of another transferential figure, paternal in this case, in Luke's unconscious. The intertransferential repetition of sibling rivalry, each of the two replaying their violent relationship with their younger brothers in their life as a couple would also be discovered in the same way.

Indeed, this mutual psychic and verbal violence would also serve as a way of avoiding any conjugal rapprochement by way of tenderness, which had a different meaning for each of them.

In fact, even if it was consciously sought after, in Luke's unconscious imagination, it signified the danger of being absorbed, even vampirised, by Corinne as he had been by his mother.

While for Corinne, tenderness had instead a twofold unconscious meaning: that of forbidden satisfaction, because she would not deserve, according to her mother, the least expression of tenderness, but rather remoteness and deprecation; and that of a dangerous incestuous *rapprochement* with her father, which she could therefore relive in the paternal transfer with Luke. On the other hand, *rapprochement* by way of this form of violence was "more bearable" on the unconscious level.

Ultimately, this form of conjugal violence seems to me to be a very costly intertransferential neurotic formation that Corinne and Luke have created and put into place, both for self-protection and to satisfy certain conflictual unconscious psychic tendencies.

An extraconjugal affair or "extraconjugal acting": A factor of crisis and/or critical symptom?

This may emerge at different times in the couple's life, in the man/or in the woman. We will most certainly look for the existence of overdetermination.

Alice, 42 years old and Jean, 55 years old, came to consult me in a rather critical state because Alice was engaging in an extraconjugal relationship that was becoming unbearable for Jean. I will develop this situation in Part II, Chapter 3,which is devoted to the technical aspects of my work.

Presence of a symptom in one of the partners disturbing conjugal functioning

We mention depression and other psychopathological troubles, behavioural troubles (alcohol, drugs), a more or less serious somatic illness, in particular.

Judith, 35 years old and Albert, 38 years old, were presented to illustrate the diverse modalities of the choice of love-object.

Presence of a symptom in a couple's child

This symptom, psychic in nature, displayed by the child can be linked to suffering in parental functioning. Thus, hostile movements may be displaced from the parental couple to the child, protecting their idealisation and avoiding the expression of unbearable ambivalence. The noisy pathology of an adolescent may sometimes be understood as a means of inciting the parents to seek treatment.

Nicole, 45 years old and Pierre, 50 years old, are the parents of Lise, 16 years old and Maxime, 14 years old.

Nicole and Pierre's conjugal life had become practically non-existent for many years and their parental functioning was conflictual. Their children were suffering considerably from this situation, each one expressing it in his or her way: Lise was showing it by a gradual disinvestment of her schoolwork leading to very worrying poor results, while Maxime was not very talkative, even falling into silence, internalising his suffering and his hostility directed against his parents. He was shutting himself up in his bedroom immediately after the family meals, smoking joints and "immersing" himself in video games.

Nicole and Pierre were very absorbed in their work. They had no longer had any erotic conjugal life for a long time and had separate bedrooms. Nicole verbalised her suffering more easily than Pierre, who readily resorted to factual, very secondarised, discourse. Nicole had always played the role of organiser of their conjugal and family life, stimulating, enterprising, expressing desires for the couple, as well as emotions and worries.

Nicole recurrently reproached Pierre for not taking interest in her and her children, therefore for not playing his role as husband-lover and father, as well as only thinking of himself, of living as a bachelor in their home and leaving her all the responsibility for their home life – something he contested. Besides her conjugal suffering, she was suffering for her children and feeling guilty about inflicting such suffering upon them. The image of their life as a couple that she was presenting to her children was unbearable for her, all the more so since, in a different way, she had also suffered from serious, enduring parental conflicts within her own family. This childhood trauma was being repeated with her own children. This was not the case with Pierre, whose personal life story was quite different, without parental conflicts, but with a great deal of independence when he was very young.

A conflictual relationship in a new couple within a reconstituted family

Mireille, 45 years old, mother of Paula, 18 years old, and Simon, 48 years old, father of Loïc, 19 years old, have had a very conflictual relationship for several years. Both divorced and parents of a child, they met shortly after they had separated from their respective spouses. Their children were very young then.

They very quickly decided to live all together. Then Mireille expressed her desire to have a child by Simon, who refused. The grief she felt would be particularly difficult to bear. While the relationship between Simon and Paula seemed harmonious, paternal, marked by tenderness and kindness on Simon's part, that between Mireille and Loïc was conflictual, even explosive. This deplorable relationship was a cause of recurring conflicts between Simon and Mireille that were invading and considerably damaging their conjugal life, all the more since Mireille reproached Simon for remaining a passive spectator, even for supporting his son and of siding with him against her.

We would come to understand that Mireille, the oldest of her siblings and her father's favourite child, had displaced the problems of a violent sibling rivalry onto her conjugal relationship with Simon and onto their new reconstituted family, principally onto Loïc. Indeed, her desire to be and to remain her father's favourite child had also been realised at the cost of the fierce exclusion and denigration of her young brother.

Simon's attachment to his son was threatening to Mireille, as he represented in her unconscious imagination a paternal transferential figure who preferred the son to the oldest daughter (in which she saw herself). Thus, within this reconstituted family, she therefore put herself in the position of a child and replayed the painful sibling rivalry of her childhood with Loïc.

Certainly, Loïc also personified Mireille's desire for a child, which had been refused by Simon. The difficulty she had had in overcoming her grief and her persistent hostility towards Simon would be displaced, in particular, onto Loïc who would carry, in spite of himself, the violence of Mireille, a maternal transferential figure and negative double of his own mother.

Simon would react to this indirectly, on the basis of their erotic life, as there he could oppose Mireille's desire, as if to punish her for the violence inflicted on his son. But we would discover that other factors were also at play.

A separation work

But these couples would also consult me to undertake a "separation work" that would be beneficial to both partners and would attenuate the inevitable suffering inflicted, not without feelings of guilt, on any children they may have.

Julie, 28 years old and André, 32 years old, parents of Bruno, four years old, came to consult me because they no longer had any conjugal sexual life. It had gradually died out after the birth of their son, Bruno. In the course of our work, the predominant sibling dimension in their life as a couple became apparent. Besides their parental couple, which was functioning fairly well, they no longer had a love life, but a tender brother-sister relationship was emerging and developing, underlain by an unconscious incestuous fantasy prohibiting an erotic life from then on. Confronted with the shared and common impossibility of overcoming this fantasy and making changes in their conjugal functioning, they decided to separate. However, they asked me to continue our work, which from then on was to help them to separate well, without making their son suffer.

Light was shed on this particularly touching request fairly quickly. In fact, Julie and André were only children of couples who had separated poorly, and they had suffered in a similar way from this situation. The experience was all the more traumatic, since not much was said about it by and with their parents, which thus plunged both of them into loneliness triggering a distressful situation. How were they to repair this traumatic experience?

As we continued to work together, we became conscious that their life as a couple also had the primordial function of finding in the other person, first of all a brother, a sister, which enabled them to no longer find themselves alone in times of distress, and finally to be able to share and face it with their masculine/feminine narcissistic double, representing then a vital source of support. It was also a matter of having a child, with the prospect, on the one hand, of repairing the damaged, wounded child who still remained in each of them and, on the other hand, of becoming good parents, much better than their own parents, so as to treat their own wounds through the child.

But becoming good parents, better than their own parents, was their unconscious conjugal contract, a triumphant oedipal fantasy that was to be operative within the framework of an offensive unconscious alliance (Kaës, 2009)[3] and that had been at least partially realised. In fact, like their parents, they separated. They therefore did not make a success of their conjugal love life. It is not very easy to make a success of one's conjugal life when one's parents did not succeed in theirs, but their failure concerned their love life and not their parental couple. This is why their success was directed towards their separation, which was above all not to repeat the trauma experienced by that of their parents, who failed on that level. Strongly identified with their son, it was therefore necessary to spare him his and their own suffering. In this way they were thus showing themselves to be good parents with their son, although their conscious feeling of guilt was patent. In addition, by identifying themselves with him, they were trying to repair their own childhood wounds.

Once they had accomplished this work, the parents left feeling more at peace and more confident, despite the wounded child in each of their unconscious minds. They decided, in particular, that each would live in an apartment near the other, with alternating custody, so as not to disturb their son's life. Their collaboration as a (brother-sister) parental couple was quite satisfactory for the comfort of their son and the child who is in them.

These consultations, early or not, attest to not only a failure of couple work but also a more pronounced contemporary concern accorded to the quality of conjugal life, as well as to the expectations and demands attending this, unprecedented in history up to now.

However, these painful conjugal situations, unmanageable by many couples, have become factors threatening rupture, which is something that we have to question ourselves about.

Notes

1 J.-G. Lemaire, *Le couple, sa vie, sa mort* (Payot, 1979).
2 J.-G. Lemaire, *Le couple, sa vie, sa mort* (Payot, 1979).
3 R. Kaës, *Les alliances inconscientes* (Dunod, 2009).

2 The preliminary interviews or the "encounter" with the couple

Making an appointment

Making an appointment with a couple psychoanalyst is, in this case, the first expression of a conjugal and individual request, which is itself the result of a certain – groupal-conjugal, intersubjective and individual psychic movement. So, one of the two partners, the woman most often, will be the spokesperson for this conjugal request, which will mainly be made by telephone, but also, more and more frequently, by email.

I propose to this partner, as spokesperson for the couple, a preliminary telephone exchange in order to clarify their individual or joint request and to discuss some practical matters.

Thus, after having invited them to explain briefly the main reason or reasons for the request, and having been informed of the source of the possible recommendation to me, I introduce myself briefly. I go on to describe my procedure of three preliminary interviews to explore their couple and its difficulties, each one lasting an hour, always in the presence of both partners, most preferably at a frequency of once a week so as to establish a good dynamic. I explain that they will be free to interrupt this process after the first or second interview, if they so desire, because at this stage no commitment has been made, either by them, or by me. In the best of cases, at the end of the third interview, I would simply tell them whether I think I can help them and, with this in mind, I would describe to them the analytic framework within which I work with couples.

Then, I inform them of fees by specifying my fee for each partner, but also for the couple, in accordance with their conjugal or personal mode of payment. Finally, I indicate to them the times when I am available, which will enable them to reflect about possibly making an appointment for the first interview, either by telephone or by email. So, we conclude this explanatory exchange, the first transfero-countertransferential aspects of which make themselves apparent, with an invitation to the partners to reflect together.

DOI: 10.4324/9781003635093-12

The preliminary interviews or the "encounter"

Some questions

J. L. Donnet has explained (2005)[1] that he uses the term "encounter" to designate the interplay between a requester and the analyst being addressed from the first time they come into contact until they reach an agreement – or disagree – about making a reciprocal commitment to psychoanalytic work. So defined, the encounter can consist of one or several interviews.[2]

Although Donnet's reflections concern individual work, they prove to be very valuable to us when it comes to thinking about not only these preliminary interviews, and what is specific to it and what is at stake in it, but also about the diverse areas of our work with couples.

Before explaining the nature and characteristics of these preliminary interviews, or of this encounter, let us join Donnet in bringing up certain underlying questions for the analyst as well as for the two partners.

First of all, these interviews take place in a particular "spot", marked by the potentiality of possible refusal, whether coming from the analyst or from the conjugal partners, and by "the deadline for responding by taking action".

For this reason, the logic of this encounter implies a conflictuality specific to the analyst that would have its equivalent in the two partners. However, the marked ambivalence of the partners always permeates these interviews, which are phobogenic and traumatogenic, because they are a source of a high level of psychic excitation that is more or less difficult to bind.

Indeed, in Donnet's words, "by suspending the representation of goal by setting up a trial situation mimicking the analytic situation, the analyst tends to bring about the emergence of the beginnings of a process",[3] which would reveal the compatibility of the psychic functioning of the virtual partners and of the couple with the analytic method.

However, and along the same lines, the analyst's listening remains more or less preoccupied with the anticipation of the act that will constitute their response, therefore, by the issues involved in a refusal to commit themselves. At this stage, therefore, the analyst is not truly in the position of being an analyst.

Consequently, these preliminary interviews represent a trial situation structurally marked by the decision, whatever it may be, that marks the end of them.

Finally, a consultative dimension is inherent in this encounter that will bring into play a third factor, the reference to psychoanalysis and its distinctive method.

Exploration of different areas of conjugal life

During the course of the three preliminary interviews usually decided upon, I proceed to a general exploration of the consulting couple that integrates, notably, its objects of suffering (complaints, reproaches, conflicts, symptoms), certain aspects of their present functioning, as well as certain critical events and stages, even traumatic ones, of their conjugal history. We also talk about the objects of mutual attraction and the expectations each one has for the other. Then each partner is asked to recount the major stages of their personal life story and the familial context within which they have lived. This is continued by enquiring into their present request regarding analytic work. Finally, we will work on detecting the first countertransferential and transferential movements.

Some characteristics of this encounter with a couple

This first phase made up of the three preliminary interviews involves many similarities with the phase of analytic work.

Indeed, this encounter is, to begin with, a transitional space-time during which the two partners meet together and can talk, talk to one another, listen to one another, listen to themselves, take the time to listen to the other person and to listen to themselves, even be obliged listen to the other person, in the presence of a third party, the analyst, something that reduces the explosive, conflictual intensity of their dual confrontation in everyday life.

Moreover, the arrangement for this encounter, within which each partner's words acquire new substance, value, even meaning, is both *doubly asymmetrical and doubly triangulated*.

This third party-analyst is consciously perceived as being a referee, a mediator. The analyst is in fact quickly invested by each partner and by the couple as a transferential mother figure, available, receptive, containing their patient's-children's suffering, placed in a sibling relationship, reviving then each partner's sibling complex in its dual, archaic and oedipal, version. But the analyst is also invested as a protective superego figure, setting limits, fair, as well as being a critic, prohibitor, observer and guardian of the consultation arrangement. That is an initial form of asymmetry and triangulation.

However, this analytic situation exposes the analyst to the regressive investment of a position of "parentified" child before a flawed parental couple in difficulty, reviving a sadomasochistic, exhibitionistic, or tender "primal scene", also satisfying their infantile voyeuristic desires. Moreover, the analyst's aloneness before the parental couple, who maintain solidarity with one another, creates another form of asymmetry, all the more so because its traumatic impact is great.

This situation, although anxiety producing, is fundamentally reassuring, re-narcissicising, individuating and subjectivising for each of the partners, restorative for the conjugal group, but also relibidinalising and relinking for the intersubjective relationship.

However, it is also eminently phobogenic, anxiety producing and a source of excitation for both the patients and the analyst, which explains, on one hand, that the couples come for consultation relatively infrequently given the extent and duration of their suffering and, on the other hand, that there are not very many analysts who work in this area.

Indeed, this encounter can reactivate the two partners' and the couple's depressive and schizo-paranoid anxieties, among them two fantasised representations, that of the *guinea pig* and that of the *spy*, identified by E. Jaques[4] (1955) can emerge. Something that he had observed among the natural groups.

Thus, the couple can fantasise that the psychoanalyst is a stranger who is not interested in the two partners for their own sakes, but because the psychoanalyst is delighted to have an opportunity to apply their method and theories. "We don't want be treated as *guinea pigs*". In addition, in coming for a consultation, the couple is experiencing a feeling of failure, reactivating depressive anxieties and anxieties of castration, of inability to manage its problems on its own. It is often experiencing a more or less conscious feeling of guilt and shame, constrained to reveal its private life to a stranger or a parental figure, therefore, to "bare itself". Moreover, the couple is apprehensive about confrontation and intervention on the part of the psychoanalyst, who could confirm its fragilities and insufficiencies, its failures, which it would prefer to deny all the same. So, this encounter with the psychoanalyst represents a genuine narcissistic threat for the couple that calls into question its own defective functioning and attacks its ideal image of itself.

On the other hand, if the couple projects its bad conscience onto the psychoanalyst and this encounter, it is then the image of the *spy* that dominates in a diffuse manner, corresponding to the reactivation of the paranoid-schizophrenic anxiety of the two partners and of the couple.

The psychoanalyst's intrusion is experienced with mistrust because it is potentially destructive, equivalent to an invasion of the "conjugal body" by the bad object.

However, mistrust circulates also between both partners because coming as a pair brings with it the danger of talking about oneself and the other person in that person's presence. It is a matter of unveiling one's psychic universe, therefore, of a potential weakening of one's system of protection. For certain people, this danger of finding out what the other person is going to say or not say about themself, about the other person, about the couple, may be great. Thus, the fantasised persecutor would also be the partner.

It may also be dangerous to verbalise thoughts, emotions, fantasies to one's partner outside of this neutral, protected space. That is why it is preferable and more reassuring to do it there. One of the risks would be the perverse use of what is said and heard as procuring a weapon for a future domestic conflict. From that point on, that place will be invested with strong ambivalence.

As I have already indicated, sibling rivalry is re-enacted within this doubly triangulated space where both partners would be seeking attention, exclusive love, narcissistic support from the parental figure represented by the analyst.

This could take the form of "phallic" competition, with the desire to be the most seductive when it comes to verbalisation, expressing emotions and fantasies and the quest for satisfaction of fantasised expectations of the analyst.

They may also seduce through suffering and engage in rivalry when it comes to its degree and mode of expression. This brings me to mention the desire of the victim, designated by the couple, to be protected by the analyst from their partner-aggressor and to induce in the analyst a masochistic identification movement as well as a countertransferential feeling of rejection and hostility towards the partner-aggressor.

One may observe a process that begins with masochistic seduction, then evolves into a perverse manipulation of the analyst causing an unconscious alliance between the victim and the analyst.

This transferential movement informs about the unconscious aspects of the conjugal bond and about the partners' repressed infantile affects.

Analysts must accept being used as an object, to be manipulated in a certain way and to a certain degree, something that will enable them, through their analysis of the countertransference, to understand certain unconscious aspects of the couple's functioning.

The analyst must also accept having this space-time of the encounter and of analytic work used by each partner and the couple as a *space for rubbish*, a place for discharge of violent affects, of fantasies of persecution and projection of internal bad objects.

Moreover, the analyst's necessary identificatory movements with each of the partners, male and female, whether the couples are heterosexual or homosexual, calls upon the analyst's bisexuality; something that requires trying and difficult psychic gymnastics.

Finally, let us view this situation as initiating the creation of a *therapeutic group,* with its specific psychic topic, dynamic and economy, which will constitute one of the agents of the evolution of the future analytic process.

Ultimately, this fundamentally traumatogenic, phobogenic and ambivalent encounter also produces multiple transferential movements determining a complex and composite countertransference that we will characterise in Part II, Chapter 3. A complex interplay of unconscious alliances will be able to be re-actualised within this transfero-countertransferential, homosexual and heterosexual, dynamic among the following transfero-countertransferential figures: father-daughter, father-son, mother-daughter, mother-son, brother-brother, brother-sister, sister-sister.

The decision to undertake analytic work with couples and its criteria

At the end of the third interview and at the conclusion of a process of countertransferential evaluation, the analyst communicates their decision to the consulting couple: "I agree to work with you, I think I can help you. I am going to present to you some rules and principles which I follow in my work with couples. It is a matter of what is called the analytic framework".

This framework will become *their* framework, once received, accepted and introjected, but also that of the *therapeutic group* that they are already beginning to constitute with the psychoanalyst.

This decision will have to take into account and to integrate heterogeneous levels of reality. On the part of the psychoanalyst, this decision therefore presupposes and implies an *evaluation*, that is to say the bringing into play of their clinical experience and of the relative anticipatory ability it enables (Donnet, 2005).[5]

Thus, the analyst's exploration of the couple will have enabled the analyst to identify in the two partners:

- their level of verbalisation and of reflexive capacities;
- the degree of investment of psychic functioning of each one, of the other and of their conjugal reality;
- their investigative drive, whose object is particularly the discovery and mastery of a meaning (M. Enriquez, 1986);[6]
- yet also an aptitude for "trusting passivation" (A. Green, 1990),[7] in which the two conjugal partners place their trust in the analyst;
- a capacity for reassessment, as the genuine individual and conjugal desire for change.

Let us finally emphasise the analyst's identificatory capacities with the two partners, the analyst's positive investment and also their anticipatory intuition of being able to accomplish good work – in short, their positive countertransference – as well as the gamble involved in forming a good *therapeutic group*.

On the other hand, if the decision is negative, the psychoanalyst will have to communicate it to the couple tactfully, that is to say, in a kind way, and simply tell them that the psychoanalytic approach may be premature or not adapted to their situation, this couple requiring a rather more interventionist and active approach of a systemic or cognitive-behavioural kind. This negative decision will inevitably be spontaneously experienced and received as a narcissistic wound, a rejection, an abandonment, confirming and reactivating their castration and depressive anxieties and the quality of bad objects that the two partners and their couple represent for the parental transferential figure embodied by the analyst. On the unconscious level, this negative decision may also satisfy the negative component of their ambivalence and thus be a relief to them. However, the suggestion of another approach is soothing and let us not forget that the potentiality of this negative decision, as much by the analyst as by the couple, or one of the two partners opposing the desire of the other, is also inherent in these preliminary interviews.

Reminder of some general characteristics of the analytic framework

The framework determines the conditions of a workspace (Green, 1990)[8] and constitutes a mute, silent backdrop, a constant allowing the variables of the process a certain amount of play. It is assumed to have an impact on the nature and organisation of the phenomena of the process, which is why the choice of framework is so important.

By its arrangement and its rules, the framework creates a transitional area within the analytic couple or the *therapeutic group* that makes it possible to provide its members with narcissistic security.

A twofold function is habitually conferred upon it: "that of superegoic, paternal symbolic *barrier* and that of maternal symbiotic *enclosure*" (Donnet, 2005).[9]

Within this analytic situation, psychoanalyst and patient occupy dissimilar positions. Certain of them are common to them, such as the rule of abstinence: by forbidding them to engage in any "real" personal relationship within or outside of the situation, it constrains them to engage in only symbolic and fantasised relationships, as well as ordinary social relationships together.

Other rules are specific to each of the two positions.

The patient's task is symbolic in nature: to express everything they think, imagine, feel in the situation, that is to say, "to symbolise" the effects it has on them as an individual. While that of the analyst is one of understanding as transference, or as resistance to transference, everything that the subject is seeking to signify in this situation and only to intervene, notably by interpretations, to help the subject understand the meaning of it (D. Anzieu, 1975).[10]

Finally, the framework implicitly contains in its definition the indefiniteness of the sequence of the sessions and the patients' possibility to bring them to an end at any time (Donnet, 2005).[11]

Stating the rules to the consulting couple

It is important to state the rules clearly and to help the couple understand them. These rules will then be the object of fantasised investments and defensive counterinvestments that will need to be interpreted. Once stated, as guarantor, the psychoanalyst will not have to make sure of their application by the couple "as a censor", but the analyst will have to seek to understand and to interpret failures to follow these rules, or the difficulties of putting them into practice.

A *first* rule concerns a set of practical indications relative to the work sessions: the imperative presence of the two partners of the couple at each session, the absence of one of them making the session impossible; the length of each session (an hour); the frequency of the sessions (preferably weekly, if not, then every two weeks); fixing a set time. "This timeslot will thus be reserved for you. You will make use of it as you can". Remember that the fee for the sessions was already specified during the first exchange.

A *second rule, the fundamental rule* of the typical cure, becomes each partner's *right, and not obligation, to say* everything that comes to their mind: what each individual is thinking, what they are feeling and what they are imagining, without being interrupted by the partner. All the while knowing that the latter will react through non-verbal, mimo-gestural and/or postural expressions, even by verbally interrupting the person speaking. With couples, it is a matter of making sure that the integrity of each one's psychic space is preserved.

Remember that Donnet (2005) considers that by proposing to the patient to say everything that comes to mind in the situation of the typical cure, the fundamental rule

> conjoins the *positive* opportunity to speak spontaneously, *freely*, and the *negative* prescription not to silence incidental thoughts ... At the same time, however, laying down the rule favors discursive and psychic eventiality *hic et nunc*; it places the session under the *virtual* aegis of free association.[12]

This rule "sets down – and rests on – the gap between '*Saying*' – which simultaneously makes saying a constraint and a freedom – and *what comes* – which refers to a heterogeneous and polymorphic psychic eventuality".[13]

This invitation to engage in unlimited freedom of speech revives in each person's unconscious both repressed desires and anxiety about transgressing the prohibition by formulating them; whence, in the beginning especially, the inhibitions, paralysis, silence.

On the other hand, in work with couples, this fundamental rule is transformed into *the right to not say everything*, therefore, the positive opportunity remains, but its negative side of not silencing incidental ideas disappears in favour of the need to preserve the integrity of each individual's psychic space. Consequently, any breaking into this space by one of the partners will be denounced and will become an object of investigation by the *therapeutic group*.

In addition, the rearrangements of the framework, according to Green (1990),[14] have no other function that to facilitate the function of representation.

In the analytic situation with couples, besides the work of verbalising affects, fantasies, thoughts and conflicts, one also finds behavioural, postural and mimo-gestural modes of expression, therefore, a sensorial and motor array, which is particularly mobilised both by the speaker and by their partner, owing to the face-to-face arrangement. Whence the great heterogeneity of signifiers (Green, 1973)[15] or modes of drive representativeness (R. Roussillon, 2008).[16]

At the same time, this rule essentially provides a certain "immunity to speech" and anticipates the fact that the latter will mobilise conflictual psychic issues, as is attested to in its formulation to the reference to objections to be overcome ("Even if that seems absurd, futile or unpleasant to you"). It therefore foresees that this conflictuality – which the method needs – will manifest itself in the activity of speaking (Donnet, 2005).[17]

If there is speech immunity, this psychic conflictuality mobilised by speech will be exacerbated in work with couples, because speaking about oneself, about the other person and about one's couple is a source of multiple anxieties, of phobic conduct and of inhibitions in the situation of the session itself and in its afterwardness. Whence "the resistances *to* saying and *by* saying" evoked by Freud.

Let me point out that this associative process will initially be able to be individual and to remain so, but it will also be able to be relayed by the partner in order to become conjugal, therefore groupal, thus expressing an eventuality that is individual first of all, then intersubjective and groupal, and therefore necessarily polymorphous and heterogeneous, which would proceed from an unconscious fantasising resonance.

The analyst is then in a position to understand the session process associatively. I will return to this in Part II, Chapter 3 (which is devoted to the technical aspects of analytic work with couples).

A third rule, that of abstinence, is common to the analyst and the couple's two partners: by forbidding them any "real" personal relationship within the analytic situation or outside of it, it constrains them to have only symbolic and fantasised relationships together, as well as conventional social relationships. This also signifies any absence of intervention into the couple's concrete reality, in the form of spontaneous personal advice and opinions on the part of the analyst or upon an "insistent" request on the part of one of the partners or the couple. Just as it presupposes the absence of individual relations on the part of the analyst with each partner. Any communication of an informative kind will always be addressed to and pertain to both conjugal partners.

Thus, by defending the integrity of our therapeutic area, we are at the same time defending the integrity of the two partners' psychic area, which we are perhaps going to restore (P. C. Racamier, 1995).[18]

From then on, the partners will leave with the freedom and the need to decide whether or not to engage in this work as a couple, which is an individual as well as a conjugal and groupal adventure.

Notes

1 J. L. Donnet, *La situation analysante* (Presses universitaires de France, 2005).
2 J. L. Donnet, *La situation analysante* (Presses universitaires de France, 2005), p. 190.
3 J. L. Donnet, *La situation analysante* (Presses universitaires de France, 2005), p. 193.
4 Cited by D. Anzieu in *Le groupe et l'inconscient* (Dunod, 1984; first published 1975); translated as *The Group and the Unconscious* (Routledge, 2014).
5 J. L. Donnet, *La situation analysante* (Presses universitaires de France, 2005).
6 M. Enriquez, "Le délire en héritage", in R. Kaës, H. Faimberg, M. Enriquez and J. J. Baranes, *La transmission de la vie psychique entre les générations* (Dunod, 1993).
7 A. Green, *La folie privée* (Gallimard, 1990); as *On Private Madness* (Routledge, 1996 (1972), inI English).
8 A. Green, *La folie privée* (Gallimard, 1990; first published 1972); as *On Private Madness* (Routledge, 1996, in English).
9 J. L. Donnet, *La situation analysante* (Presses universitaires de France, 2005).
10 D. Anzieu, *Le groupe et l'inconscient* (Dunod, 1984; first published 1975); as *The Group and the Unconscious* (Routledge, 2014, in English).
11 J. L. Donnet, *La situation analysante* (Presses universitaires de France, 2005).
12 J. L. Donnet, *La situation analysante* (Presses universitaires de France, 2005), pp. 8–9.
13 J. L. Donnet, *La situation analysante* (Presses universitaires de France, 2005), p. 66.
14 A. Green, *La folie privée* (Gallimard, 1990; first published 1972); as *On Private Madness* (Routledge, 1996, in English).
15 A. Green, *La folie privée* (Gallimard, 1990; first published 1972); as *On Private Madness* (Routledge, 1996, in English).
16 R. Roussillon, *Le jeu et l'entre-je(u)* (Presses universitaires de France, 2008).
17 J. L. Donnet, *La situation analysante* (Presses universitaires de France, 2005).
18 P. C. Racamier, *L'inceste et l'incestuel* (Les éditions du Collège, 1995).

3 The work and its technical aspects

I am now going to elaborate a discourse on the questions of the method, of the site and of the analysing situation, of the transferential levels, of the associative processes, of the listening and of the interpretation, while referring at times to the individual arrangement, at times to the group arrangement, so as better to situate, differentiate, characterise and particularise our work with couples, so little known in its singularity and in its identity.

Method of individual work and with couples

J. L. Donnet (2005)[1] considers that the matrix of the analytic method is *the free association–interpretative afterwardness pair*, the correlate of which would be the fundamental postulate of the processual dynamic flowing out of the transferential encounter, a dynamic that on all its levels activates the psychic representing.

In addition, free association reveals regressive thought in images, especially visual ones, but the obligation to speak obstructs this tendency, so that the material thus produced is useful in interpreting and becoming aware. Speech then functions as counterinvestment, and its narrative level seems to situate it outside the associative process. Whence, according to Donnet, the antagonism between imaging thought and speech.

The method only ever deals with representations, with speech phenomena viewed from the angle of their "transferential addressing value".

This method thus requires *transference onto speech* – with its vicissitudes. We expand upon this aspect later in the chapter.

Of course, face to face and in the presence of a couple, we also have to deal with signifiers other than speech, such as mimo-gesturality and the postures of the individual speaking, and those of their partner, who is listening and reacts through these non-verbal signifiers.

From another perspective, Donnet deems that "in the same way that it unites and separates the patient and the analyst through its reference to a third factor, the method joins and disjoins theory and practice by situating itself on its interface".[2]

DOI: 10.4324/9781003635093-13

For his part, P. Denis (2010) has looked at the ethics of the psycho-analytic work that would base itself on the method itself and its applica-tion, that is to say, more on the implementation of the means of the cure than on what may result from it. Moreover, analysis of the psycho-analyst's countertransference is necessary as a condition and ethical requirement of the psychoanalytic method. It is found even "at the heart of psychoanalytic ethics".[3] Which very obviously continues to be valid in our work with couples.

Site, analysing situation and analytic situation

Donnet differentiates between the *analytic site* and the *analysing situation*: "The analytic site contains everything constituting the offer of analysis, including the analyst on the job", while "the analysing situation results unpredictably from the sufficiently adequate encounter between the patient and the site. It implies the subjectivated use, as found-created, by the patient of the resources of the site and of their singular configuration".[4]

Thus, sites are going to organise themselves on the basis of the diverse work situations proposed in the field of psychoanalytic practice, such as that with couples. They display sufficient consistency and typicality, their own logic and produce their own processual dynamic. In addition, the analysing situation leaves its mark on the specific functional unity constituted by the patient-analyst situation as a whole consisting of a unity of liaison between the patient's intrapsychic processes and their exteriorisation on the scene of the transference, on the one hand, and, on the other hand, between the psychic processes of the two protagonists, to the point of creating through the interplay of the transference and the countertransference an analytic couple, a chimera (M. de M'Uzan, 2005),[5] a shared play area.

Thus, the analytic situation of the individual cure would result from the:

> antagonistic and complementary interplay of two scenes, the unity of which *ultimately* lies in the fact that the transference onto speech required by the method can operate on two levels, intra- and inter-subjective [...]:

> - *An intrapsychic scene* in which the inner discourse can use words as perceptual organs exploring the inner world [...].
> - *An intersubjective scene,* in which the most specific thing at stake is relative to the *setting into action* of the transference through speech [...]. But the characteristic of the scene is that it displaces onto the analyst alone the issues surrounding the fundamental rule and its function as a third factor.[6]

What about the group psychoanalytic arrangement?

The group psycho-analytic arrangement is pluri-subjective, and R. Kaës (2015)[7] points out that this morphological specificity involves several consequences, in particular regarding the nature of the associative regime and discourse.

First of all, each participant and all the other participants are in a position to respond in the presence of and to the presence of every other one.

If, in the cure, the associations are *successive* and *addressed to the analyst*, on the other hand, in the group, the associations are *successive* and *simultaneous*, they are *interdiscursive* and *interfering*.

In other words, each subject's associations encounter the associations of another, or of several other subjects, therefore are connected both with the goal-representations that are proper to each subject, and that polarise their associative discourse, and with the associations of the others.

In addition, in the cure, the subject cannot simultaneously be on the level of the primary process and on that of the secondary process, while these two levels co-exist in the group.

Based on this double reference to the individual cure and to work with the groups, what can we say about the site, about the analysing situation, about the arrangement with the couples and about its implications?

Adopting Donnet's formulation, I can say that the analysing situation concerns the "sufficiently adequate" encounter of the two partners, of their couple, as a group, and this specific site.

In order to characterise this site and this analysing situation with the couples, let us immediately point out that they involve a face-to-face groupal arrangement.

Indeed, work with couples is a face-to-face arrangement that in fact shares certain distinctive features of individual therapy that are proper to it, therefore different from the typical cure, and that combine with those of the groupal arrangement with couples. Let us look at them right now.

First of all, being face to face maintains the exchange or the avoidance of eye contact. It integrates into the reciprocal communication or into its modalities of drive representativeness, the motor and sensorial levels, with the mimicry, gestures, postures particularly called upon and invested that are the diverse pathways of the flow of excitation, but also sources of excitation and of fantasised activation inducing multiple anxieties and defence mechanisms in the protagonists.

The radical bringing into play of the fundamental rule is rarely possible. If analysts attempt to preserve the associative functioning and interpretative afterwardness, they do not however have at their disposal a temporality analogous to that of the classic analytic site. Here, the analysts' relationship to their management of time is rather different: they are led to intervene more often, and their decisions to intervene or to interpret are made more rapidly.

Donnet (2005)[8] considers that all these phenomena are connected with the uniqueness of the session, as in couple therapy: "The process of the single particularly invested session urges on to the creation of a sample of analysis that is pertinent in its own right".[9]

Moreover, being face to face is rather supportive of the relationship to the analyst *in person*, the perception and representation of whom are inseparable.

Consequently, less favourable for grasping transference as such, being face to face raises the question of the difference between the transference and *the relationship* in an analytic situation.

C. Parat (1982)[10] considered that if the typical cure facilitates transference, being face to face rather uncovers *the relationship* corresponding to the patient's investment in the person of the analyst, an investment tinged with trust. This investment is based, on the one hand, on projective, subjective elements, a spontaneous link having a positive tone, and, on the other hand, on objective elements perceived by the patient from the time of the early contacts.

We, in fact, find all these aspects in our work with couples and, in particular, the investment tinged with trust in the person of the analyst.

Let us continue further with Donnet's mode of investigation and reflection.

The analysing situation with couples would imply the subjectivated use by each of the partners, and the conjugal use by the couple-group, as "found/created" of the resources of this site and of their singular configuration.

It would result there from the antagonistic and complementary interplay of *several scenes*, the unity of which would rest on the fact that the *transference onto speech* can operate on the *threefold intrapsychic, intersubjective and groupal plane*. We will also find *a transference onto the motor-sensorial level*.

Thus, we could establish that this whole formed by the two conjugal partners, their couple, the analyst and the situation constitutes a functional unit, that is to say, a unit of liaison between:

- Each partner's intrapsychic processes and their exteriorisation on the scene of the transference onto the analyst, which correspond to each individual's intrapsychic scene.
- Each partner's psychic processes and those of the analyst creating an individual analytic relation.
- The two partners' intrapsychic processes and their exteriorisation within their intertransferential relationship, which corresponds to their intersubjective scene, which in turn expresses certain connected or "combined aspects" of their infantile neurosis.

- The psychic processes of the conjugal group and their exteriorisation onto the scene of the transference onto the analyst, which corresponds to an initial groupal scene.
- And also between the psychic processes of the two partners, those of the conjugal group and those of the analyst, forming then a *therapeutic group*, through this complex play of multiple transferences, and of the analyst's composite countertransference – something that corresponds to a second groupal scene.

Drawing inspiration now from Kaës' reflections, we can say that the analytic situation with a couple is a plurisubjective groupal situation. Consequently, each partner's associations will encounter those of the other and connect with them. They will be able to be successive, but also simultaneous, interdiscursive and interfering when they have a dialogue in the presence of the analyst. Thus, a groupal discourse formed of conjugal associative chains will be the expression of their conjugal group and of its shared and common formations.

Let us also add that, in the couple, the two levels, primary and secondary, co-exist.

Let us explore other aspects

Since the analytic situation induces a *regression*, a whole part of the analytic process rests on it, the aspects of which are multiple, just as a part of the countertransferential attitude is organised in terms of this regression. It will inevitably be narcissistic in nature, but also pregenital and oedipal in nature, particularly giving rise to phobic attitudes and movements.

Indeed, P. Denis (2010)[11] has emphasised that the analytic situation imposes on patients recourse to an "auto" activity that requires them to let go of different elements of the outside world in order to invest their own psychic functioning, inner objects, something that reinforces their narcissism.

However, the analytic situation with the couples also requires of them an investment of the partners' psychic functioning, something that relibidinalises the intersubjective relationship, as well as an investment of their groupal functioning, which tends to reinforce conjugal narcissism.

Let us also mention the *phobogenic dimension* of the analytic situation with the couples based on Denis's reflections on individual work.

On each partner's side, and on that of the couple, there exist phobias about both the framework and the transference onto the analyst – even though this transference is not as great as in the individual cure – as well as about the intertransferential relationship, those of a voyeuristic and exhibitionistic nature: baring oneself in front of the partner, the analyst, disclosing one's own psychic functioning, that of the partner and of the couple, for example.

Certain behaviours on the part of patients, such as tardiness and frequently missing sessions, as well as the quasi-mutism, or frequently interrupting the individual speaking instead of listening quietly, would be in response to a phobic movement.

Observable on the analyst's side is the fear of the patients, with the phobia of being an object of control by each partner, but also the fear of the couple, reactivating either a sadistic primal scene, traumatic in nature, or an overly arousing erotico-tender one that becomes the object of movements of exclusion, envy and jealousy.

Additionally, there is the phobia of exercising control over patients, and of everything that would be perceived as being aggressive.

Behind these fears generally looms, as Denis suggests, a phobia of the transference of the patients, of their virtually massive movements, as hostile as they are erotic, experienced dangerously, but also in return, the phobia of the power invested in the analyst that can be exercised abusively with and over the patients.

Let us also mention a possible phobia of silence, of any retentive and marked attitude of neutrality; which can induce excessively numerous interventions, a tendency to respond to direct questions instead of interpreting the transferential movement that gave rise to them.

Finally, this analysing situation with the couples induces *a certain type of functioning of the psychism of the partners and of the couple, as well as symbolisation.*

The therapeutic group

Let us go back to the therapeutic group produced by, and specific to, the analytic situation with couples and expand upon certain of its economic and dynamic aspects.

Recall that the *therapeutic group* is composed of the analyst, the two partners forming the couple and the conjugal group, who are bound by diverse unconscious alliances that are as structuring as they are defensive.

Thus, we can detect a basic structuring alliance, on the one hand, between the analyst and each partner, and, on the other hand, between the conjugal group and the analyst, who are situated in the transfero-countertransferential field.

Their function would be to constitute a limit, a restraint and to favour the processes of representation and symbolisation.

A fundamental dimension of this basic alliance is grounded in the love of transference-countertransference (Kaës, 2009).[12]

As for the two conjugal partners, they are united by offensive and defensive, structuring alliances constitutive of their conjugal group. Certain of them will therefore be particularly mobilised in the dynamic of this *therapeutic group* in structuring, defensive and offensive form.

In addition, defensive alliances, alliances of resistance to the analytic process, can be established between each partner, or between the two partners and the analyst, which will manifest themselves in shared symptoms or in *acting out*. They will vary in accordance with the processual moments of the work, therefore, and be inherent in the countertransferential and transferential manifestations.

Yet, invested as a fantasised and libidinal object by the two partners and by the couple, as well as by the analyst, the *therapeutic group* is also the place of the reactivation of the originary fantasies in its members, among which we can find: the intra-uterine fantasy corresponding to the group's imaginary space in work session and suggesting the interior of the protective and containing maternal body; this three-person situation of the *therapeutic group* easily reactivates the primal scene fantasy, something that permits all the possible permutations of it; as well as the seduction fantasy with its forms of heterosexual and homosexual coupling, arousing movements of rivalry, envy and jealousy and mobilising each partner's sibling complex; finally, the castration fantasy can express itself through themes of inadequacy, impotency, deficiency or loss.

On the economic plane, this *therapeutic group*, upon which the processual dynamic of our work in part depends, will be an object of differentiated investments, on the part of each partner and of the couple, of a sublimated homosexual, aim-inhibited, erotic, narcissistic nature, but also markedly ambivalent in nature, depending on the times and periods of the work. On the analyst's part, this group will also be invested in a sublimated homosexual, aim-inhibited, erotic, narcissistic mode.

However, the work of the death drive (A. Green)[13] in the two partners and within their couple will also manifest itself in diverse manners, in particular, to resist change, even to undermine the analyst's work, leading to a feeling of stagnation (of "turning around in circles", of "not going anywhere"), despite considerable effort, and even more than that to the premature interruption of our work.

The work of the analyst and their psychic functioning with couples

The analyst's countertransference

Tackling the subject of the work of analysts and their functioning necessarily requires that we look at their countertransference, which will determine, in particular, their modalities of investment and of listening to their patients, to their associations, but also their identificatory abilities, their comprehension, their multiple interventions, as well as their interpretative activity.

So, we begin with some reflections by P. Denis and M. Neyraut.

Denis (2010)[14] considers countertransference as first of all being the transference of a transference that therefore makes reference to the analyst's pre-existing transferential experience.

He sees countertransference as "the space itself which presents itself to the expression of the transference. It contains it, permits its implementation or, on the contrary, limits it or disrupts its movement".[15]

The active, central, positive element conferring upon it its psychoanalytic specificity and maintaining it, is therefore, according to Denis, an attitude of receptiveness to the expression of the patient's unconscious movements and the goal-inhibited libidinal investment of their psychic functioning besides conditioning its dynamic value.

Countertransference is also an instrument of investigation and interpretation of the patient's transferential movements.

Paradoxically, the attitudes habitually called *countertransferential reactions* are reactions of the analyst inherent in the fleeting or more lasting investment of their patient, as an ordinary person and not of their psychic functioning; which would attest to resistance to their countertransference.

For Neyraut (1974),[16] an analyst's countertransferential thought, which is considered to be at work during an analyst's involvement in an analytic situation, also designates the analyst's ideas, fantasies, representations, whether induced or prior to a sequence. If their countertransference refers to analytic theory and thought in general, "this thought and this theory acquire personal specifications delimiting a particular field of listening".[17]

He also conceives of countertransference as a protective shield that can be prior to the drive solicitations revealed by the transference as well as being consecutive. It is most often consecutive and triggered by the transferential manifestations revelatory of objectal drive motions that it attempts to oppose.

In our work with couples, the countertransference of the analyst, who forms a *therapeutic group* with their two patients and their couple, will be complex because it is composite, a space of receptivity to the transferential movements of each partner and of the conjugal group.

Just as with regard to this *therapeutic group*, the object of a transference of a groupal nature, the analyst will develop a *groupal* countertransference.

From these fundamental bases, we can explore some areas and characteristics of the analyst's work.

The communication between the two partners, that of their couple and the analyst's work of intervention and interpretation is situated in this "transitional field", the potential space between them and us.

With Green (1990), we can say that the analyst's inevitably conflictual work – a "product of a constant battle between the hearing, the poorly heard, the unheard and the unhearable [...]",[18] in particular – is always fundamentally *work of thinking and of representing the psychic processes* at work in each of the partners, in their intersubjective relationship and within their conjugal reality.

Green also invites us to observe that *negative hallucination* is not absent in this work; it corresponds to all the times in which the analyst does not understand anything about the material, can neither represent it, nor discover the connections in it.

What about analytic listening?

Within the framework of the typical cure, Neyraut[19] defines two fundamental modes of this listening: concordant listening and discordant listening.

This concordance or this discordance refer to the effects of harmony or of disharmony in the patients' and the analyst's flow of associations.

Kaës (2015)[20] considers that in the group situation listening is determined by different and specific epistemological positions.

He personally advocates a *polyphonic listening* based on an epistemological position that conceives that

> the Unconscious produces its effects, makes itself heard, not only in the space we select, but in another, as is its habit. I am taking into consideration here three psychic spaces which coexist and interfere in the group situation and whose associative chains are interwoven in three discourses. Is such polyphonic listening possible? Can the relationships among these three spaces be the object of simultaneous, and distinct listening?[21]

What are the conditions and modalities of this?

This polyphonic listening would first of all depend on the analyst's capacity to perceive and to conceive this threefold source of the specificity and relationships of the associative processes, while being aware that they cannot hear *everything* that is said in these three spaces and in the relationships among them.

On the technical plane, by relying on the analysis of the groupal psychic apparatus's processes of functioning, Kaës detected two categories of *knotting points* between these spaces, the phoric subjects and the unconscious alliances, which thus condense the psychic reality of the three spaces.

The phoric subjects are those subjects who perform phoric functions in the group: these are the spokespersons, the dream-bearers, the symptom-bearers, ideal-bearers, the scapegoats, for example.

It is a matter of the co-productions of each subject, both in their singularity and in their relationship to the group.

> Bringing this specialized ear's attention to the place occupied by the phoric subjects and the unconscious alliances in the transferences and in the associative process makes it possible to hear not only what each individual signifies in the group, but also what he or she signifies for

another and for more than one other, and what is signified and heard by all of the participants in the group.[22]

And with couples?

Our listening to patients as couples is one of a polymorphic and plural associative discourse referring also to "the heterogeneity of the signifiers", to use Green's expression (1973).[23] We will then have to be "polyglots" (Green, 1990).[24] Just as polyphonic listening is obligatory given the three structuro-functional levels I have defined.

We therefore have to listen to each partner's associative discourse, that of their intersubjective relationship, which is intertransferential in nature, but also that of their conjugal group when the meeting of their associative chains will form a groupal discourse.

We also need to be sensitive and attentive to the effects of agreements and disagreements between each partner's flow of associations and between those of the partners and those of the analyst, in particular. We strive to detect the knotting points represented by the phoric subjects and the unconscious alliances within this conjugal configuration.

Let us emphasise that this associative and transferential clinical material involves significant traumatic impact on the analyst, who can sometimes feel overwhelmed and exhausted.

The identificatory capacities of the analyst

However, there is no listening without identification; whence the need to address the identificatory capacities called upon in the analyst during the session.

And, first of all, what pertains to primary identification, as numerous authors have emphasised.

Indeed, stating the fundamental rule, therefore, the invitation to engage in free association, mobilises the primary identification processes to constitute in the analyst a common world of representations and affects with the patient.

To hear the other person, to understand, to feel what the other person feels, must not one be capable of becoming this other person at times?

Starting from this fundamental disposition, composed of unconditional openness to the patient's psychism, the analyst's capacity for hysterical identification steps in to allow them to espouse the patient's movements from time to time, all the while preserving sufficient personal mobility to extricate themself from it.

Analysts can sometimes feel stuck, without any possibility of representation, in an archaic identification, something that will come to indicate to them in afterwardness that their psychic field is the target of a projective identification of their patients.

What about the analyst's secondary identifications in the integration of their psychic bisexuality?

The work of analysts relies on their receptive, even passive, and feminine identifications that are called upon; that is to say, on their capacity to let themselves be permeated with their patients' strange (because foreign) representations and to familiarise themselves with them so that they can become introjectable objects.

The handling of the interpretation, into which intrusive speech brings its nourishing value, embodies the range of paternal and masculine identifications.

All these identifications are necessarily mobilised in any work with couples, be they heterosexual or homosexual. However, it is the complexity of all these identificatory processes that dominates owing to the plurality of the objects of investment present.

What about the analyst's psychic economy?

First of all, *let us distinguish between two objects of investment in every patient: the person of the patient and their psychic functioning* (Denis, 2010).[25]

The person of the patient is the object of a plural libidinal investment.

The patient's psychic functioning is the object of an aim-inhibited libidinal investment, which relies on the narcissistic investment of the analyst's functioning during the session, and also on the investment of the analyst's work and method.

Following C. Parat (1967),[26] I can add that associated with this is a sublimated homosexual investment, any professional activity corresponding to the "world of others" of the oedipal organisation of the genital stage.

With couples, the analyst will be confronted, on the one hand, with the person of each partner, with their couple as a group, and, on the other hand, with each one's psychic functioning and with that of their couple. Whence a plural libidinal investment having a high energy level, with its traumatic dangers, that the analyst will have to master with the help of an efficient protective shield system. Which explains a fairly frequent state of fatigue following sessions.

As for the analyst's unconscious psychosexuality, it is particularly called upon in the course of individual work and more so with couples.

Let us look at orality, with the analyst's need to be nourished by the associations of the two partners of the couple, as well as the pleasure of nourishing patients with interventions and interpretations. We can mention the analysts' voyeuristic desires, which are stimulated by the present representation of a couple resonating with primal scene and seduction fantasies.

We also encounter their investigation drive with the desire to know and to understand, therefore, to seek and grasp a meaning.

Moreover, their anality, with its sphincterian function of opening and closing, will contribute to selecting the non-verbal, associative and verbal material of the two partners and of the couple. Anality and its active-passive pair contribute to determining the mode of listening. And we should not forget the desire for mastery and control as well as their tenacity.

The castrated-phallic pair is also mobilised with its times of potency and of impotence, when analysts are confronted with certain situations arousing a feeling of triumph or of incapacity, of failure, and therefore of castration. Finally, let us repeat that their psychic bisexuality will manifest itself in their capacities for identifications, feminine as well as masculine.

Fundamental conditions and tactical aspects of work with couples

Psychoanalytic work with couples, which is inevitably situated in afterwardness, represents a transitional, intermediary space-time between the couple's suffering, corresponding to a failure of their couple work, and, on the one hand, the discovery of their conjugal psychic functioning and that of each partner, on the other hand, the occurrence of beneficial changes finally made possible by obtaining the means favourable to carrying out much more satisfying couple work, which will have positive effects on the two other, sexual-bodily and sociocultural, conjugal realties.

I consider that if the strategy of psychoanalytic work with couples is based, on the one hand, on the interpretation of these multiple transferential movements – proceeding from the analyst's composite countertransference, and, on the other hand, relating to the three levels of their psychic reality (individual, intersubjective and groupal), this work necessarily involves fundamental conditions and tactical aspects, something that we are going to examine now.

The double use of the "well-tempered" silence, not only of the analyst, but also of the conjugal partner who must listen without interrupting their partner

In the individual cure, according to B. Grunberger (1971),[27] silence aims to constitute a "narcissistic union" with the patient enabling the patient to restore their wounded narcissistic integrity. It therefore involves a narcissistic restorative function of the patient. Indeed, the respect and restoration of the patient's narcissism are fundamental elements of any analytic process.

Silence also places emphasis on the patient's own psychic activity as driver of the cure, helping to preserve the autonomy of their processes and their subjective appropriation (Donnet, 2005).[28]

If silence has two meanings, that of void and that of verbal abstinence, in every case, the latter must be connected with the intense work of elaboration in which an analyst engages during their silent listening. A component of the framework, the analyst's silence is connected with other parameters defining the analytic situation. The reason for silence in analysis is to make the emergence of *representation* possible (Green, 1990).[29]

It becomes something like a backdrop against which associative thinking unfolds, just as it "constitutes the backdrop against which the patient's projective figures are going to move (or be moved), take shape, be written down, be composed. It would be a something like a prerequisite of interpretation".[30]

However, in our work with couples, the analyst must "play" with the silence and the distribution of speech between the two partners in order to favour the function of representation and the processes of symbolisation in them.

A facilitation of the common verbalisation of thoughts, affects and fantasies

We will facilitate the common verbalisation of thoughts and affects underlying the conflicts and the symptoms, as well as the expression of fantasies and their circulation – which corresponds to the partners' interpretative activity – by inviting each of them to say what they imagine about the partner's psychic reality and about the conjugal reality.

Indeed, for that, it will be a matter of establishing a reassuring narcissistic framework and of inspiring an investment of trust in the person of the analyst, something that will help both partners overcome their resistance to speaking and their phobia of revealing their inner world, in particular. They will thus be able to verbalise and exchange their thoughts, their affects and their fantasies, then confront them with situations of daily life as well as with events of their personal and/or conjugal lives.

This verbalisation in common will mobilise their preconscious and favour expansion in particular.

Distributing speech between the two partners and supporting the succession of individual and conjugal associations

It is the job of the analyst, master and guardian of *psychoanalytic playing* (M. Parsons, 1999, cited by Donnet, 2005),[31] to distribute speech between the two partners while safeguarding the speaker's discourse and keeping the listener silent and attentive. The analyst will also be able to allow the two partners to associate between themselves, permit them to engage in free circulation of words, affects and fantasies, as long as unconscious resistances are not detected. Indeed, certain so-called "free" associations serve the resistances articulated as a couple. A groupal process is then at work. This is why, when the analyst can identify them, they must interrupt their conjugal associative process and inform the partners of it. Then the analyst can lead them to reflect upon this and together discover a meaning in it.

Ultimately, with couples, analysts must constantly *play flexibly* between two attitudes, active and passive, in the service of the session's processual dynamic.

Helping to "reformulate" and to elucidate certain contents expressed, that is to say, to accord value to what is verbalised and to help in expanding upon it

PATIENT: "I was very surprised and disconcerted when I learned it ..."
ANALYST: "You were very surprised and disconcerted ... Could you be
    more precise and expand upon this?"

This tactical aspect has a narcissising function for the one speaking, but also a function of stimulating their function of representation and symbolisation, as well as of mobilising the investment of their partner's listening, even of stimulating their investigation drive and of libidinalising their bond in the session.

"Lending" representations and affects if necessary, that is to say, temporarily offering an "auxiliary Ego" to one of the partners, even to both

According to P. Marty (1990),[32] and this is particularly so with psychosomatic patients, exercising a *maternal function*, which rests on the *maternal possibilities of the therapist*, whether a woman or a man, is required and consists of "an accompaniment, which is above all, but not exclusively, verbal, accompanying, following or barely preceding the subject's states and movements".[33]

Analysts will thus offer their own elementary systems of sensitivity, of representations, of behaviours, possibly of rudimentary defences, and will progressively play the role of deficient functions in their patients.

This is valid and justified with certain conjugal partners who prove deficient when it comes to verbalising fantasies and affects.

Thus, when I ask one of the two, usually the man, the following question:

ANALYST: "What do you feel while listening to what your companion is
    telling us, what does it do to you?"
PATIENT: "I think that ..."
ANALYST: "I am not asking you about what you are thinking right now,
    but about what you are feeling, about your emotions".
PATIENT: "I don't know ..."
ANALYST: "I am going to help you: does that surprise you, astonish you,
    sadden you, or anger you, or rather worry you; or amuse you then,
    please you ...?"

PATIENT: "I would rather say that that astonishes me and saddens me".
ANALYST: "So, that astonishes you and saddens you. Were you able to imagine that, madam?"

Thus, these work sessions with certain couples are going to help certain of the partners, the men usually, to develop their fantasising and symbolising skills, therefore, their preconscious, through the intervention of their partner and of the analyst, who will in fact play a maternal role by temporarily "offering" them an "auxiliary Ego".

Linking and symbolising interventions prior to interpretative activity

It is a matter of the essential operation of the linking.

Instead of letting the film play out or the associative thread unwind, the analyst will at times intersperse the discourse with interventions connecting together the "bits of the discourse" (Green, 1990).[34] The goal of the connecting thus performed is, therefore, to reconnect the disconnected elements in order, at a certain point, to interpret and no longer just intervene.

Green has pointed out (1990):

> There are two phases in symbolization, [...] the first connects the terms of the conscious, the second uses the connections established to connect them with the split unconscious. This work of connecting and reconnecting thwarts the work of the destruction drives. To be effective, it must be superficial. The goal of this work on the *surface*, on the level of associations, is to constitute a preconscious which does not usually fulfil its function as mediator or as filter in both directions between conscious and unconscious.[35]

Something that is also accomplished with the couples, reconnecting the "bits of discourse" of each of the partners, then connecting them together, constructing a conjugal discourse so as to activate and develop each partner's preconscious and that of the couple.

Interpretative activity

Some areas of the transference

Before addressing the specificities of the transferential manifestations with couples, I would like to recall briefly some areas of transference in individual work that will prove highly useful to us, then some particularities of the transferential manifestations in the group situation.

In the typical cure

On the part of the patient, *dynamic transference* implies an *investment of neutrality*, that is to say, the possibility of experiencing the analyst on all possible levels, which requires a comparable attitude on the part of the analyst: a dynamic countertransference able to accept all possible transferential expressions (C. Bouchard, 2000).[36]

However, this attitude implies recognition of the analyst's otherness and an implicit distinction between their person and their function, between the analyst object of transference and the analyst interpreter.

Negative transference represents an "overly" hostile or "overly" erotic "monovalent" transference, which arrests the movement of the analytic process and freezes the cure in an "immobile movement" (Denis, 2010).[37]

As for *lateral transference*, it opposes transference insofar as it exports repetition onto another object and into another space.

If, in the session, in the here and now, transference expresses something that has happened elsewhere and in the past, lateral transference expresses outside of the session, onto another object, the transference carried out on the analyst.

It in fact seeks to avoid excesses in the here and now, whence its function of economic regulation that its movements of lateralisation fulfil.

Not forgetting the *transference onto speech* required by the method and its vicissitudes, such as instances of *acting* through speech as modes of expression of resistance *to saying*.

Donnet deems that

> *acting through speech* [...] seems to accomplish – and even to signify – the neutralization of what is at stake in speech, and to do that to the extent of including the saying of transference in it. It results from this that the speech is addressed to the analyst in person in a direct, *operational*, mode reflecting thought with a concrete appearance. There is neutralization – in the drive sense – of/in the transference onto speech.[38]

In the patient, this can attest to a phobia of their mental functioning, but also to a negativity. The *acting through speech* interrupts the associative flux.

From the beginning of a session, the patient says to the analyst: "What are the dates of your next vacations?" Or, in the course of a session, after a period of silence during which a patient especially invests their sensoriality in the service of the observation of the objects of the analyst's office: "Is this little sculpture new?"

But also, following a telling about a fragment of a dream: "What do you think of my dream, doctor?" or "How must I understand my mother's attitude?" or "What should I do?".

The patient turns away then from their inner world, from their own thoughts, in order to invest sensorially the elements of the analyst's material setting or psychically what is happening or is supposed to happen in the analyst's mind, or else, what they are projecting onto the analyst.

Specificities of transferential manifestations in groups

The group is the site of the emergence of particular configurations of transference.

Kaës takes up the four transferential objects identified by his colleague A. Bejarano (1972):[39]

- The central transference of each member of the group onto the psychoanalyst, who would function as an archaic paternal imago or as a prohibitor oedipal imago or an idealised and benevolent imago.
- The groupal transference onto the group as an object of drive investments and of unconscious representations.
- The lateral transferences onto the members of the group as sibling imagos.
- The transference onto what is outside the group (the external world, place of projection of individual destructivity and place of hope.)

The first three of these objects of transference are found in couples.

In addition, the unconscious psychic objects are transferred at the same time or successively into the group, depending on each participant's transferences and the development of the groupal process, while they manifest themselves successively in the individual cure.

Just as the other members of the group, the psychoanalyst is the object of successive or simultaneous transferences of several subjects and is not the *only* object of the transference.

In addition, in the group situation, Kaës (2015)[40] finds, we are dealing with a twofold process of *diffraction* and of *connection* of transferences. He says:

> the diffraction of the transference is the regime that prevails in the group. The diffraction of the objects of the transference onto all the members of the group, onto the group and onto the analyst, that is to say, onto the objects predisposed to receive them in several psychic places, is not a dilution of the transference, but an economic distribution of the drive charges attached to these objects.[41]

However, the objects and places of transferences are also *interconnected*.

What about our work with couples?

Everything that has been brought up about various areas of transference in individual work, as well as about the specific features of transferential manifestations in groups, is quite obviously valid and highly valuable in my work with couples, but with some very marked particularities.

First of all, let us recall that this face-to-face arrangement serves rather to support the relationship to the analyst *in person*. Consequently, being face to face is less propitious to getting hold of transference as such. Whether it be that of each of the two partners or of the conjugal group.

As in the group arrangement, we will find a diffraction and a connection of objects of transference.

Depending on the phases of the therapy, a difference of transferential investment of the person of the analyst may exist between the two partners, while the conjugal group will have and will maintain its own transferential investment, also variable in accordance with the periods of the work with the analyst.

As for the intersubjective relationship between the two partners, I have maintained that it is partially constituted of intertransferential movements constitutive of an intertransferential neurosis repeating and permitting the reconstruction of certain aspects of the partners' infantile neurosis. It is also involved in the diffraction and connection of objects of transference.

There will, therefore, be a reciprocal and multiple transferential investment of the imagos embodied by each one, be they maternal, paternal or sibling, in particular. This investment is to be differentiated from that of their own person, in their subjectivity and their identity.

What can be said about this in the course of therapy?

This intertransferential neurosis displays itself, lets itself be seen and heard, in the presence of the analyst who will react to it with their specific countertransference, which is different from the countertransference in response to the transference of each of the partners and to that of the conjugal group.

In addition, as in the individual face-to-face arrangement, although analysts strive to preserve associative functioning and afterwardness, they do not have at their disposal a temporality analogous to that of the individual cure. Their relationship to time is modified and they are led to intervene more often. As *masters of analytic playing*, their interventions will also be dictated by the need to distribute speaking between the two partners, all the while leaving them the freedom to engage in exchanges with one another, at the risk of forgetting the voyeuristic and attentive presence of the analyst. "They put on a show in the presence of their analyst".

Regarding the diverse forms of transference onto the two partners speaking and acting through speaking, some clarifications prove necessary.

Indeed, the fundamental rule is modified in our work with couples, because the obligation to say everything is replaced by the freedom and the right to say everything along with the possibility of keeping things for oneself, in oneself, in the presence of the partner. It follows from this that the conflictuality involved in saying inevitably proves to be lessened. However, at least two other major and fairly regular conflictualities manifest themselves there.

The first is inherent in the partner's presence, potentially anxiogenic and inhibiting, a source of resistance *to saying* what comes to mind, both for the analyst and for their partner.

The second is tied to the individual work undertaken by one or both partners. They do not know whether they can or must express in their space-time of the session together as a couple, certain thoughts, affects, childhood memories, fantasies in relation to their personal lives that spontaneously come to mind and that they consider that they have to reserve for their individual work, therefore, for *their* analyst. Just as they may hesitate to communicate certain aspects elaborated or certain discoveries made in the individual session, with a whole underlying transgressive dimension, even one of betraying *their* analyst.

Regarding acting through speech, I think that, on the one hand, the face-to-face arrangement mobilising motor and sensorial investment, and, on the other hand, the modification of the fundamental rule act in its favour, with everything that this implies. As well as the constant comparison and the difference of investment between individual work, its space-time and that of working as a couple, with elements of lateral transference from one towards the other and reciprocally.

Finally, on the topic of the dynamic and economy of the *therapeutic group* and of the plural transference of the two partners and of the conjugal group onto this group, we have already looked at the unconscious alliances and the originary fantasies reactivated. However, this *therapeutic group* will also represent one of the motors of our work with couples, and its evolution will depend, in part, on its sublimated homosexual and narcissistic investment and its dynamic animated by plural conflictualities.

I also wish to mention an observation occasionally made concerning certain couples in which one of the partners could never engage in lasting individual work, having interrupted it one or several times, with diverse psychotherapists. Then, they finally *found* (*rediscovered?*) this arrangement of working as a couple, therefore, in the presence of their partner, which proved to be much more satisfying. I translate this as being narcissistically reassuring and comforting. This partner's regressive needs probably required a maternal presence that would revive the mother-child dyad enabling them to satisfy fusional-symbiotic needs and narcissistic completeness.

Another hypothesis could be that this partner perhaps could not tolerate a single object of transference in individual work but this groupal arrangement of working together as a couple enables them to diffract their transferential movements, something that is less traumatic on the economic plane, and therefore less disorganising and less anxiogenic.

Many patients will never undertake individual work, but will however *use* and benefit from working together as a couple, in the presence of their partner, in order to accomplish individual work at the same time, something that also incorporates my conception of work with couples. This makes the groupal arrangement a felicitous opportunity for these patients.

Characteristics of our interpretative activity

Remember that our interpretative activity will concern the three structuro-functional levels, intrapsychic-individual, intersubjective and groupal; and, in addition, that in particular it will present certain specific features connected with transferential configurations and the particularities of the associative process and of interdiscursivity.

On each of these levels, our interpretative activity will be able to reveal the diverse modes of the expression of the failure of the two partners' couple work.

On the groupal level

On the groupal level, we will be able to identify, on the one hand, on the basis of the two partners' interdiscursive, successive and/or simultaneous verbal associations, and of their non-verbal signifiers – underlain by their individual psychic processes that will therefore express themselves in the groupal process – and, on the other hand, on the basis of some conjugal transferential movements, something that expresses their conjugal unconscious psychic reality, that is to say, what is *shared and common* to them, whether verbalised or not by "*we*".

We think, *we* feel, *we* imagine, *we* want to have a child, *we* plan to buy an apartment, *we* want to end our therapy.

Thus, as Kaës (2015) clearly expresses it,

> the interpretation points to the shared and common constructions, and especially those which are at the origin of the suffering or of the pathogenic conflicts of the whole, such as they result from the processes and formations of the intersubjective tie and of the whole. Among these common constructions, I accord the greatest importance to the pathogenic and defensive unconscious alliances.[42]

Indeed, our work to interpret this *conjugal material* will enable us to bring the couple to discover certain unconscious fantasies, organisers of their conjugal reality, certain of their shared and common anxieties, their offensive and defensive, even pathogenic, unconscious alliances that underlie shared symptoms, certain phoric functions borne by one of partners, and also shared and common resistances. Just as certain aspects of their conjugal culture will reveal themselves as their discourse proceeds.

On the intersubjective level

Our interpretative activity will also concern the *varied modalities of their intersubjective relationship*, within which their systems of object relations are revived regarding their pregenital and narcissistic dimensions, as well as their sibling and OEdipus complexes linked. All these elements partially constitutive of their intertransferential neurosis will enable us to reconstruct with both partners some fragments of their infantile neurosis that they have shared. But also to initiate elaborative work.

In addition, we uncover some of their structural conflictualities.

On the individual level

On this level, I consider that this site and this analysing situation specific to work with couples both offer each partner the opportunity to accomplish personal work in the presence of the other person. In addition, we have found that the reciprocal investment of each partner's life story and psychic functioning, one of the objects of our work, therefore, the discovery of certain aspects finally verbalised of their psychic life (their unconscious life especially), can foster personal and intersubjective rearrangements through the suppression of representations, affects and fantasies produced and maintained by the other person over the course of time, then proving erroneous after confrontation with the partner's psychic reality that has been revealed. We also endeavour to explore relationships of each partner's ego with the love-object and with the couple-object, to detect in particular the nature of the anxieties and of the correlative defences mobilised, as well as the conflictual relationships between these two objects.

However, we encounter and must always confront along the way, whatever the time, the period, the modes of expression and the levels of intensity, the two major enemies that, according to Green (1990),[43] thwart our capabilities and our work: this is the combination of repetition and of destructivity.

Alice and Jean

This example of interpretative activity, which concerns the two levels, first individual, then intersubjective, is determined by a specific transfero-countertransferential dynamic that effectively ruled out taking the groupal level into consideration.

Alice 42 years old and Jean 55 years old came to consult me in a rather critical state, sent by a sexologist whom Jean was consulting. Alice was engaging in an extraconjugal relationship that was becoming unbearable for Jean because, according to him, it was not supposed to have evolved the way it has.

Some historical and biographical elements

About the couple

Alice and Jean met 20 years ago in Paris during a dinner with friends. Alice was then 22 years old, an attractive beautician living in Belgium. Jean was 35 years old, a wine merchant, divorced, father of one child for whom he was not the guardian – he was very well off in those days. For him, it was love at first sight, which was not the case for Alice, who experienced this first meeting differently. Nonetheless, she was attracted to this reassuring, very intelligent, generous, reliable man, upon whom she could lean. For Jean, Alice was such a beautiful woman: apart from her sensuality and her intelligence, he was moved and touched by her sensitivity and her fragility.

Their relationship began very rapidly, with Jean plying Alice with gifts and talking of love. They settled down together very quickly. About their life as a couple, Alice expressed certain reservations, but nevertheless accepted it. She would nonetheless continue to feel a great deal of ambivalence, the hostile component of which would remain unconscious and well counterinvested. Alice soon expressed the desire to have a child, something to which Jean was not at all opposed. So it was that Jules was born, then Claire, three years later, and Alice devoted herself fully to them, at the risk of losing her autonomy. They experienced years of very happy conjugal and family life – theoretically. Stepping back, Alice became aware of a certain alienation both in her relationship with her husband and in her family life, something that caused her to enter into a period of profound personal and conjugal crisis. And Jean experienced serious professional difficulties accompanied by a sharp drop in income.

As a family, they left France for Canada where Jean tried to get his feet back on the ground. He succeeded partially, but the crisis in their relationship was severe and profound. Alice brought up the idea of separating, a thought Jean considered unbearable to the point of wishing to commit suicide. They consulted a couple therapist and then began therapy, which they interrupted prematurely. After some years, they returned to Paris, but the conjugal crisis persisted and intensified. Having taken up her studies again some years earlier, Alice became a nursery school-teacher. She quickly found a job in a childcare centre, while Jean found himself jobless and in a very precarious financial situation. It was within this context that Alice brought up the desire to have an extraconjugal relationship. The meeting of her lover, "authorised" and "offered" by her husband was to be subject to the condition that it was to be purely erotic and of short duration. However, this extraconjugal relationship, which unexpectedly lasted longer, worsened their crisis even more. This situation. which he was unable to control, was very painful for Jean, and wounded him narcissistically. He asked Alice to bring it to an end, but she was against that and could not do it. She felt lost, indecisive, torn between the pressure of her husband and the perverse manipulations of her lover, whom she also used as a means of detachment, emancipation and decision-making power with regard to her husband's domination of her. It was within this context that they came to consult me, and, for Jean, one of the objectives of this therapy was the interruption of the extraconjugal relationship and the "reintegration-recuperation" of Alice into the couple.

Alice

Alice was born in France, the older of two children, with a brother two years younger than her. Her mother quickly fell ill and was frequently hospitalised in the mental hospital for depression. Alice was quite young when her father abandoned them. Faced with this situation, the two children and their mother left for Belgium to live with the children's maternal grandmother, who would play a major role in their childhood and adolescence., taking care of her grandchildren because their mother was incapable of it. But this grandmother was controlling, and the way she dominated Alice became unbearable. Alice left this pathogenic family environment, a source of multiple dissatisfactions and dangers, as soon as possible. After secondary school, she studied to be a beautician by taking odd jobs. She also met various men, without any desire to live together as a couple until she met Jean. Alice's life with Jean and her desire to be a mother would therefore repair the little girl greatly harmed by her primary parental deprivations having determined early narcissistic traumatisms that still had not been worked out. The anti-depressive function of the couple and of motherhood proving obvious.

Jean

Jean's father was a Jew of Polish origin who was deported to a concentration camp during the Second World War. Presented both as a hero and a womaniser, he treated Jean badly, which made him an object of great ambivalence. Jean's mother is described as uninteresting, distant, not very affectionate. Jean was the middle child. His two brothers for the most part acquired satisfactory professional situations. After taking university-level courses in business and enology, Jean became a prosperous wine merchant. However, he had suffered from a lack of love on the part of his mother and violence on the part of his father, who Jean admired as much as hated. However, Jean and his first wife separated fairly early and he became single again, not wanting to remarry.

The structuring of Alice and Jean's couple and intertransferential neurosis

Alice and Jean's meeting was therapeutic, having a principally reparative and anti-depressive purpose. It was probably the principal object of their defensive unconscious alliance or denegative pact (Kaës, 2009).[44] For both of them, it was a matter of repairing through the love-object and through their couple, traumatisms, sufferings and deficiencies – of an essentially narcissistic nature, having produced depressive affects.

What also brought Alice and Jean together was an unconscious hatred of the parent of the opposite sex transferred onto the partner and highly counterinvested by erotic and tender motions (impulses, or affects). As well as hatred directed towards the parent of the same sex.

They are also driven by a shared and common oedipal fantasy of triumph over defective parents consisting of being better parents than theirs were, as well as a better husband and wife, suggesting the constitution of an offensive unconscious alliance (Kaës, 2009).[45]

Interpretative activity and transfero-countertransferential dynamic

Alice and Jean had found themselves in such a state of distress that they assigned me the role of "emergency couple therapist".

"Warmly recommended by a sexologist", to use Jean's expression, I was already, and from the start, invested as "a very good professional", suggesting a highly positive, even idealising, individual and conjugal transferential movement from the time of the first interview, one determining basic trust and high expectations for a caring attitude and narcissistic benevolence.

Jean told me very early that he had seen certain of my lectures on the internet, which he had particularly liked.

I represented both an idealised protective, solid transferential father-figure and a receptive, benevolent mother-figure. So, it was easy for me to imagine the occurrence of future hostile movements, in particular, in the case of disappointment or reactivated narcissistic wounds.

The ambivalence of the intensity of their transference in fact manifested itself very quickly and was the cause of just as highly ambivalent countertransferential movements in me, which contributed to making our sessions difficult, characterised by a state of growing tension in the course of each one of them. Consequently, they conditioned my interpretative work to the point of playing a role in the tempo, style, structuro-functional level of the couple's psychic reality and in the content of my interventions, which were then received by Alice and Jean in an ambivalent sense, marked by gratitude, admiration, but also by reticence, even criticism and protest. Here is an exemplary illustration of the interpretative process proceeding out of my countertransferential movements.

Jean regularly "gobbles up" all the time for speaking at Alice's expense, something that forces me to interrupt him over and over again and with a certain amount of difficulty. Curiously, Alice does not seem to want to interrupt him to express herself and thus take advantage of the space of time that is legitimately hers. I then presume the existence of an "unconscious conjugal alliance" (Kaës, 2009).[46] In doing so, "he forces me" regularly to overrun the amount of time allotted for our sessions. I gradually begin to feel overwhelmed by the unending, continuous verbiage that accompanies his spellbinding gaze, thus exercising a hold on me. My tension and irritation are all the greater since I am trapped by the rule of free association, which in this case is obviously at the service of both individual and conjugal latent resistances.

His need to use up all the time devoted to each session – which, he explains, he prepares for and moreover awaits impatiently – gives me insight into the nature of that need, both intertransferential, of a sibling kind, and transferential, of a motherly type. It is a matter in this case of reviving an aspect of his sibling complex and of a mode of anal object relation to his mother. Indeed, as in the family environment of his childhood, he has a need in our sessions, in my receptive, benevolent maternal presence, to capture my attention at his wife's expense, within the framework of a painful, fierce, sibling rivalry. This situation arouses very ambivalent countertransferential attitudes and affects in me. They are combining with those passively experienced invasive, controlling ones, in particular, that have informed me about certain invasive aspects of Jean's conjugal behaviour with Alice and the way in which she might experience it, as well as the highly sadistic-anal dimension of their intersubjective relationship. Alice reacts to this by adopting defensive attitudes of mockery, therefore of disguised hostility.

All the while, the affects of solicitude, irritation and injustice I feel with respect to Alice enable me to picture to myself the lack of consideration from which she might have suffered.

However, behind this transferential and intertransferential mastery exercised by Jean, and beyond my countertransferential irritation, I perceived and imagined infantile distress in him combined with a marked masochistic component connected with a sadistic component that I sensed in Alice.

Having detected these transfero-countertransferential games fairly early, I am all the same regularly led to have to interrupt Jean in order to give Alice a chance to speak. So it is that I told Jean about a long *individual* interpretation, which I had put off and reflected upon in order to find the least narcissistically wounding and most understandable way to put it into words. Indeed, my countertransferential movements *forced* and *led* me to the individual level then to the intersubjective level, so ruling out the group level of their couple. In addition, let us mention my academic style that is also countertransferential in nature. I finally said,

> I have wondered for some time about your need regularly to monopolise the conversation during our sessions and I imagined that, in the present situation, in that I represent a mother figure from your childhood, for your unconscious imagination, you need to have my

exclusive attention – at the expense of your wife, placed then into the position of a sibling – because you certainly suffered from the lack of it due to the fact that you quite obviously had to share it with your siblings. Moreover, I was also thinking that by obliging me to interrupt you over and over and persistently so, in this attitude, you all the same put yourself in the position of the child who is going to get himself punished both by a frustrating mother figure and by a violent father figure.

Moved and seeming rather relieved, Jean responded: "What you say makes sense to me. Moreover, in my family, I was considered the 'ugly duckling'". The wounded child in him touches and moves me.

This situation makes apparent an unconscious distribution of roles, within which Jean plays the "bad patient/bad son", while Alice enjoys the narcissistic advantage – repairing old, open, wounds – of being in my eyes a transferential parental figure, a "good patient/good daughter", the better of the two "transfero-countertransferential siblings", which is accompanied by a sadistic pleasure expressing itself in a little derisive smile.

Then I ask Alice: "How do you feel about your husband's need to spend so much time talking?" "I'm used to it, so it doesn't surprise me", she answers with a slight smile in a weary tone of voice.

She did not in fact say what she was feeling, as if, in her family situation, there was no room for Alice to verbalise her own feelings, as here, in our sessions, in my presence and in that of her husband.

In fact, I understand that Alice is re-experiencing quite old frustrations and injustices, just as Jean is, in this manner, expressing his need for exclusive love, that which his parents and siblings deprived him of.

The afternoon following our morning session, feeling upset, he called me, to tell me that his father had beaten him violently on numerous occasions. I listened to him kindly while reminding him that it was one of the principles of the context of our meetings that everything had to be recounted during the session and in the partner's presence, so what he was telling me would then have to be recounted during the next session. This transgressing of the principles of our framework confirms the image he has of himself and his role of "ugly duckling" within the couple, reflecting his position within his family.

Let us now discuss the expectations and benefits associated with our work.

Expected effects and benefits

Donnet has looked at the *necessary autonomy of the method* that postulates that the consistency of the therapeutic effects will depend on the rigour with which one will have been able to implement the method. "The method's functional autonomy resides in both the fact that its purpose must not be determined and in the virtual presence of its (psycho)therapeutic vocation".[47]

Donnet distinguishes between the specific psychic transformations inherent in the process that are directly tied to the method and the expected healing made of the indirect effects at a distance from these psychic transformations.

Psychoanalytic healing can only be evaluated through the conjunction of specific transformations *and* their effects in the patient's life.

What would be the psychic transformations inherent in work with couples? What would be the indirect effects of it at a distance which would correspond to the said "additional" healing?

First of all, work with couples revitalises, re-dynamises each partner's couple work, and does so right from the beginning. Something that will have an impact on the three conjugal realities, psychic, sexual-bodily and sociocultural.

On the groupal level

Our work fosters a rearranging of the shared and common formations, such as the defensive alliances, pathogenic ones in particular, a suppression, attenuation or an acceptance of the shared symptoms, but also of certain phoric functions, as well as a fantasised reorganisation, and a redistribution of investments among the shared and common objects, and the separate and individual objects, in particular.

On the intersubjective level

Work with couples will make it possible to:

- achieve a genuine "unsticking" of each of the partners by decreasing the excessive identificatory movements, those of a projective and adhesive nature in particular, thus favouring a process of individuation/separation, then of subjectivation in them, as well as a re-narcissisation finding expression in greater autonomy;
- lower the level of structural conflictualities, and tend towards less rigidity in their intersubjective relationship leading to making it more flexible, to its re-libidinalisation, to improved fantasising and affective circulation – lessening ambivalence and freeing tenderness, for example – and finally to more open distribution of the roles alternatively played by each one (father, mother, child, brother, sister, friend);
- rearrange certain aspects of the intertransferential neurosis through interpretative work that will aid, let us remember, in the reconstruction of the two partners' infantile neurosis and to the elaboration of infantile conflicts in the presence of the partner in this privileged situation of afterwardness.

On the individual level

Let us stress the fact that working together as a couple is also individual work in the presence of the partner, which will foster individual psychic transformations having an impact on both the intersubjective relationship and on the conjugal reality. However, our work will facilitate the acceptance of a certain degree of dependence on and of invasion by the love-object as well as by the couple-object, and it will also bring about an evolution of the representations of the love-object and the couple-object, becoming then more integrated into the world of inner objects and, therefore, less invasive. Furthermore, these changes will be able to motivate one or both partners to undertake individual work.

The effects of this psychic work will inevitably manifest themselves on the levels of sociocultural, sexual and bodily reality, as well as in family, if it is a matter of a parental couple and social life.

The improvement or the resumption of an erotic life may accompany this evolution, but this is not a certainty. Investment of the bodies may evolve, showing itself in greater reciprocal caring, seduction and concern.

The couple will bring up, in particular, rearrangements (economic and dynamic) in the family, the repositioning of each one within the family group, the re-establishing of clear boundaries between the parental couple and the children. Just as it will talk about changes having occurred in its "work couple" inducing rearrangements in its professional, domestic reality, even in its varied social relationships.

However, the evolution may be less patent, more limited, sector specific, owing to the existence of multiple, still irreducible resistances.

Finally, certain couples decide to separate in the least heartbreaking manner possible, successfully or unsuccessfully, yet "knowing fully what they are doing".

On determining the end of the sessions

Remember that the framework implicitly contains in its definition the indefinite duration of the sequence of the sessions and the possibility for the patient to end them at any point.

Determining the end of the sessions is an *act* taking place in reality and so constituting a decisive reintroduction of the act into a situation to a large extent based on excluding it (Donnet, 2005).[48]

Whatever the modalities of doing this may be, it must be looked at as a form of *taking action* proceeding in two phases: The phase of determining the end of the sessions through a verbal exchange, the effects of which will be able to be elaborated upon during the remaining sessions; and the phase of terminating the sessions, the elaboration of the effects of which requires the actual absence of the analyst.

The entire analytic situation is then modified since an essential element of the framework has disappeared: the indefiniteness of the sequence of the sessions. The period beginning at the time of the inaugural act is limited in length and planned, and a whole work of separation and of mourning is going to begin enabling the patient to limit the traumatic dimension of the termination.

The most usual manner of proceeding is that the analysand fixes an endpoint – in the near future or deferred – and that the analyst confirms that decision.

What about the couples?

The couples may spontaneously mention their desire to stop during a session by announcing that it will be the last session for diverse reasons – in particular, stagnation, boredom, one partner's desire to stop as opposed to the other partner, who wishes to continue – or they act to interrupt our work by a telephone call or an email.

In the best of cases, we can begin to discuss this prospect of ending our work, then think about it. The resistances can then manifest themselves by forgetting to think about it, the conjugal anxiety about termination therefore reactivating a conjugal anxiety about separation, even about abandonment by a parental transferential figure who would be bored with their children experienced as unsatisfactory, as "bad children", not responding to the fantasised expectations of a parent.

We therefore set an endpoint together and we keep to it.

The work thus evolves towards this cut-off point, bearer of ambivalence, mixing relief, satisfaction and separation anxiety, fear of finding oneself alone and having to cope with things alone, as before. The work of mourning can thus begin.

Notes

1 J. L. Donnet, *La situation analysante* (Presses universitaires de France, 2005).

2 J. L. Donnet, *La situation analysante* (Presses universitaires de France, 2005), p. 38.

3 P. Denis, *Rives et dérives du contre-transfert* (Presses universitaires de France, 2010), p. 177.

4 J. L. Donnet, *La situation analysante* (Presses universitaires de France, 2005), p. 19.

5 M. de M'Uzan, *Aux confins de l'identité* (Gallimard, 2005).

6 J. L. Donnet, *La situation analysante* (Presses universitaires de France, 2005), pp. 76–77.

7 R. Kaës, *L'extension de la psychanalyse* (Dunod, 2015).

8 J. L. Donnet, *La situation analysante* (Presses universitaires de France, 2005).

9 J. L. Donnet, *La situation analysante* (Presses universitaires de France, 2005), p. 163.

10 C. Parat, "Transfert et relation en analyse", *Revue française de psychanalyse*, 46, 2, (1982), pp. 357–364.

11 P. Denis, *Rives et dérives du contre-transfert* (Presses universitaires de France, 2010).

12 R. Kaës, *Les alliances inconscientes* (Dunod, 2009).

13 A. Green, *Les chaînes d'Eros, l'actualité du sexuel* (Odile Jacob, 1997).

14 P. Denis, *Rives et dérives du contre-transfert* (Presses universitaires de France, 2010).

15 P. Denis, *Rives et dérives du contre-transfert* (Presses universitaires de France, 2010), p. 31.

16 M. Neyraut, *Le transfert* (Presses universitaires de France, 2008); first published 1974).

17 M. Neyraut, *Le transfert* (Presses universitaires de France, 2008); first published 1974), p. 41.

18 A. Green, *La folie privée* (Gallimard, 1990), p. 396.

19 M. Neyraut, *Le transfert* (Presses universitaires de France, 2008; first published 1974).

20 R. Kaës, *L'extension de la psychanalyse* (Dunod, 2015).

21 R. Kaës, *L'extension de la psychanalyse* (Dunod, 2015), pp. 181–182.

22 R. Kaës, *L'extension de la psychanalyse* (Dunod, 2015), p. 184.

23 A. Green, *Le discours vivant* (Presses universitaires de France, 1973).

24 A. Green, *La folie privée* (Gallimard, 1990).

25 P. Denis, *Rives et dérives du contre-transfert* (Presses universitaires de France, 2010).

26 C. Parat, "L'organisation œdipienne du stade genital", *Revue française de psychanalyse*, 31, 5–6 (1967).

27 B. Grunberger, *Le narcissisme* (Payot & Rivages, 1993; first published 1971).

28 J. L. Donnet, *La situation analysante* (Presses universitaires de France, 2005).

29 A. Green, *La folie privée* (Gallimard, 1990).

30 A. Green, *La folie privée* (Gallimard, 1990), p. 373.

31 J. L. Donnet, *La situation analysante* (Presses universitaires de France, 2005).

32 P. Marty, *La psychosomatique de l'adulte* (Presses universitaires de France, 1990).

33 P. Marty, *La psychosomatique de l'adulte* (Presses universitaires de France, 1990), p. 96.

34 A. Green, *La folie privée* (Gallimard, 1990).

35 A. Green, *La folie privée* (Gallimard, 1990), p. 395.

36 C. Bouchard, "Peut-on interpréter le transfert négatif?", *Revue française de psychanalyse*, 64, 2 (2000), pp. 383–393.

37 P. Denis, *Rives et dérives du contre-transfer* (Presses universitaires de France, 2010).

38 J. L. Donnet, *La situation analysante* (Presses universitaires de France, 2005), p. 74.

39 Cited in R. Kaës, *L'extension de la psychanalyse* (Dunod, 2015).

40 R. Kaës, *L'extension de la psychanalyse* (Dunod, 2015).

41 R. Kaës, *L'extension de la psychanalyse* (Dunod, 2015), p. 173.

42 R. Kaës, *L'extension de la psychanalyse* (Dunod, 2015), p. 184.

43 A. Green, *La folie privée* (Gallimard, 1990).

44 R. Kaës, *Les alliances inconscientes* (Dunod, 2009).

45 R. Kaës, *Les alliances inconscientes* (Dunod, 2009).

46 R. Kaës, *Les alliances inconscientes* (Dunod, 2009).

47 J. L. Donnet, *La situation analysante* (Presses universitaires de France, 2005), p. 147.

48 J. L. Donnet, *La situation analysante* (Presses universitaires de France, 2005).

Concluding reflections and perspectives

We have now arrived at the end of our journey, which began with a reminder about the concept of couple work, work of a specific nature, undertaken within the three conjugal realities, psychic, sexual-bodily and sociocultural. Before exploring the topical, dynamic and economic aspects of couple work on each of the three structuro-functional levels of the conjugal psychic reality regularly stimulated and nurtured by certain authors, I considered it pertinent to discuss love and being in love, as essential components and *primordial time* for every couple, then to reflect upon the structural times and fundamental unconscious psychic organisers that contribute to the construction of every couple, whether heterosexual or homosexual. Something that leads us to raise questions about the conditions, determinants and modalities of the choice of the love-conjugal partner, that is to say, its historicity and the work undertaken, namely the psychic work of choosing a partner, corresponding to an individual compromise formation, but that will become intersubjective owing to the construction of an intertransferential neurosis repeating the infantile neurosis of the two partners in afterwardness. The dimension of satisfaction of a plural – narcissistic, erotic, tender and aggressive – nature involved was evident, while its defensive dimension, which clearly contributes to making the love bond last over time, therefore in a conjugal reality, was new. The innovative work of J.-G. Lemaire[1] made a great contribution here.

The common denominator in going from the work of choosing a partner to couple work, then to working with couples, reveals itself to be *work*, *psychic work* in this case. This psychic work that Freud never ceased mentioning, starting with dreamwork, but about which he also spoke as the third component of the definition of the concept of drive in 1915: "[…], as a measure of the demand made upon the mind for work in consequence of its connection with the body".[2]

This work, which is work of binding to start with, then of unbinding and of transformation, bearer of rebindings, thus runs throughout Freud's works as a central theme. It has also run throughout our book, to the point of constituting its own central theme of it also. Why?

DOI: 10.4324/9781003635093-14

Because this concept of couple work, from which all conjugal functioning proceeds, has in fact enabled us to propose and develop a metapsychological approach to the psychic reality of the couples in connection with its three continually interrelating structuro-functional levels. Just as it played its role in conjugal temporality, of a plural nature, and its vicissitudes.

However, as with all work, couple work involves failures, which manifest themselves in diverse ways, among which figure, in particular, different forms of suffering to which we are exposed as couple psychoanalysts. Whence the need arises for work with couples which must, in particular, revitalise the couple work failing in the conjugal partners. This work with couples proves difficult and uncertain, because it is complex, owing to its multiple aspects and dimensions.

We have tried to highlight some specific features of our work with couples through comparisons with individual work, on the one hand, and, on the other hand, with the arrangement for working with groups. Among these specific features, we have identified, in particular, the *therapeutic group* – composed of the two partners, the conjugal group and the analyst – as one of the agents driving the analytic process with couples.

It is a matter of being modest in one's ambitions with couples, but also endowed with a good masochism, guardian of life, in order to be able to bear up and keep going.

In addition, if we have offered some elements of a response to the two-fold question of how and why individuals form a couple, as well as to that concerning the conditions of keeping that couple psychically alive, we have also brought up questions associated with elaborating a reflection on the separation of the two partners and the breaking-up of the couple.

However, another question immediately comes up: is the couple a goal in itself? Must one form and live as a couple in order to blossom, to be fulfilled, to "live happily", as they say?

Is it recommended for everybody? Would it present dangers for certain subjects? And what types of dangers for what types of subjects?

What would be its advantages and its inconveniences?

"In this respect, one must *guard against a dangerous contemporary mystification which would extol the virtues of living as a couple as a social and personal remedy*", wrote Lemaire (1979).[3]

> No matter how important it is and how interesting studying it is from a clinical or scientific point of view, *the couple cannot be considered as a goal in itself*. It is a very specific kind of group having a distinctive mode of functioning with its advantages and its inconveniences. Advantages for its members as long as they are bound by implicit or explicit feelings of love and for the family which comes from them.[4]

But it has its inconveniences and can have pathogenic effects. "Pathogenic for its members, the couple can also be so also for those around it".[5]

These issues surrounding advantages and inconveniences lead us to the present-day fact of the growing number of single persons, both "primary" and "secondary", in our Western society, then to another question: how are unconscious psychic determinants of this major contemporary phenomenon, unprecedented in history up until now, to be explained from a psychoanalytic perspective?

In fact, I would like to take advantage of the opportunity to bring up some questions now regarding the psychic determinants and conditions of the contemporary choice to remain single, tolerated and even favoured by our society. Something that will enable me to make the transition from my present book towards an upcoming one about singlehood using a pluri- and interdisciplinary approach integrating history, anthropology, sociology and psychoanalysis, as I did in *The Couple: A Pluridisciplinary Story* (2016).[6]

One distinction, which is not rigorously juridical in nature, is in any case necessary: that between "primary" singlehood and "secondary" singlehood, that is to say between subjects who have never experienced conjugal life and those who have experienced conjugal life through one or several experiences of living together, or not living together, institutionalised by marriage or not. They may be divorced or widowed.

Starting from this fundamental distinction the psychic determinants differ.

Indeed, "primary" single persons, who therefore have never had any conjugal experience, perhaps have a terrifying unconscious fantasised representation of the couple suggesting a stifling, closed, even absorptive, invasive or devouring space, reactivating in them a persecuting, omnipotent archaic maternal imago. They then take on a rationalised protective posture of avoidance through demands of independence and freedom from all sorts of obligations and social and family pressures.

Is it a matter of "fragile subjects" for whom conjugal life could obviously constitute some dangers, given its regressive aspects in particular?

In this regard, let us remember that on the fantasised level, the love relationship reactivates the tendency to mutual fusion, to erasing the boundaries between two subjects, an attempt to re-form the symbiosis of the mother-child dyad.

In addition, a double process of partial annexation by the other person and of the other person and of reciprocal possession is at work, with their correlative share of alienation and loss of freedom.

However, conjugal love also associates narcissistic enrichment and confirmation with aggressive, tender and erotic satisfaction.

If one of the priorities of these single persons, whose psychopathological difficulties would be of a *borderline* or identity-narcissistic kind, is in particular to preserve their blurred, fragile psychic borders, as well as to protect themselves from their anxieties of separation and intrusion, they could nonetheless construct a conjugal organisation characterised by a distance between the two partners' psychic spaces, thus constituting a "transitional space" and a limitation of the density of their relationship to the detriment of the pleasure sacrificed.

If it is essentially a matter of fighting against an individual's own over-flowing, therefore, disorganising inner destructivity, something that represents one of the couple's fundamental psychic functions, within the framework of this defensive strategy, the couple then appears to be the mode of organisation of these mutual projections and introjections by which each individual, confronted with their own destruction drives, uses the other as a source of external support for both good and bad inner objects.

Forming a couple is a way of getting ridding of or of metabolising each partner's depressive and/or paranoid tendencies.

So, why remain single when an individual is so fragile and could benefit from certain advantages offered by a conjugal organisation protecting them from these multiple psychic dangers?

Considering now the oedipal organisation of the genital stage described by C. Parat (1967),[7] we could say that these single persons live in a two-way rather than a three-way system, thus pregenital and non-oedipal. Without a relationship said to be heterosexual with a conjugal partner, even a homosexual one, they only have left to them the narcissistic investment of their person and that of the "world of others", object of a sublimated homosexual investment.

And what about "secondary" single persons?

They have had one or more conjugal experiences that had been able to offer various kinds of benefits, but also that constituted an alienating, fragilising, and therefore potentially traumatic and disorganising, even desubjectivating, dimension in the form of pathogenic unconscious alliances.

The compulsion to repeat these traumatic experiences is no longer functioning in these subjects, they have chosen a protective solution in this new status of "secondary" single person. This solution represents a mod-ality of reconstruction and of identity safeguard, but also of major narcis-sistic reinvestment and subjective reappropriation of their psychic life, and of their life quite simply.

On the level of the oedipal organisation of the genital stage, these secondary single persons would have proceeded to regression towards a pregenital organisation favoured by points of fixation. Will it prove to be temporary or definitive? The drive economy is so mobile, even unforeseeable ...

We could envisage other questions and other beginnings of responses, but have decided to leave things here for the time being and so to lay all that to rest, a time of latency being necessary before the elaborative after-wardness of the upcoming book.

Notes

1 J.-G. Lemaire, *Le couple, sa vie, sa mort* (Payot, 1979).
2 S. Freud (1915), "Instincts and their vicissitudes", *The Standard Edition of the Complete Psychological Works of Sigmund Freud*, XIV (Hogarth, 1966), pp. 121–122.
3 J.-G. Lemaire, *Le couple, sa vie, sa mort* (Payot, 1979).
4 J.-G. Lemaire, *Le couple, sa vie, sa mort* (Payot, 1979).
5 J.-G. Lemaire, *Le couple, sa vie, sa mort* (Payot, 1979), pp. 343–344.
6 É. Smadja, *Le couple et son histoire* (Presses universitaires de France, 2011, in French); as *The Couple: A Pluridisciplinary Story* (Routledge, 2016, in English).
7 C. Parat, "L'organisation œdipienne du stade genital", *Revue française de psychanalyse*, 31, 5–6 (1967).

Index

mystification, protection 150
mythical tales 69

narcissising function, tactical aspect 132
narcissism 47, 48; extraction 70;
   objectality, antagonisms 96, 98;
   primary narcissism 60; secondary
   narcissism 60
narcissistic completeness 137; source 14
narcissistic contract 66; relation 70
narcissistic double 22; imagos/figures,
   fixations 23; specular narcissistic
   double 23
narcissistic element 80–81
narcissistic failure 18, 21
narcissistic foundations, reorganisation
   70
narcissistic fragility 98
narcissistic framework 131
narcissistic identifications 61; Ego,
   relationship 41; mobilisation 21
narcissistic integrity: reassurance 9;
   restoration 130
narcissistic investment 11–12, 36;
   grounding 68; impact 32; mobility
   43; receiving 86; work object 38
narcissistic libidinal currents,
   unbinding 18
narcissistic nature, accomplishment 38
narcissistic object 78; choice 53; choice,
   integration 26; mutual co-identification 53
narcissistic reparation, modality 98
narcissistic security, providing 115
narcissistic wounds 14, 76–77;
   reactivation 72
narrative level 119
natural life cycle, dynamic 76–77
negative transference 134
negativity: negation 59; repression 67
neuroticising potentiality 55
neurotic nature, symptoms 71
neutral field, presence 60
neutrality, attitude 124
new couple, conflictual relationship
   106–107
new objectal relation, creation 41
Nirvana principle, compulsion 75
nonerotic life, libidinal movements
   (impact) 49
nostalgia, phase 14

object: attachment 76; choice, modality
   27; choices (Lemaire) 25–28;
configuration 65; creation 37; defensive choice 26–27; Ego, partial fusion
   45; impact 37–38; inadequacy 18;
   metapsychological couple drive
   object 32–33; persecutory interiorised
   objects (external support), partner
   choice (impact) 27; positive
   characteristics, correspondence 25;
   relation, modes 86–87; relationship
   44; representations 34–35; roles
   34–35; symbolising/subjectivating
   functions 34; transference 137; unity,
   constitution 35–36
objectal environment 33–35
objectal failure 21
objectal investment 36; mobility 43
objectalising function 42, 48
objectality 47, 48; narcissism, antagonisms 96, 98
objectal libidinal currents, unbinding 18
objectal relations, evolution 76
object relations: constellation 56;
   economic aspects 42–43; facts 40–42;
   systems 40–44; transference,
   relationships 41–42
oedipal child, guilt 86
oedipal conflict: impact 56; involvements 18; positive oedipal conflict 53
oedipal desires, repression 26
oedipal fantasies 11
oedipal fixation 20
oedipal hatred, heir 47
oedipal internal objects 35
oedipalised sibling complex 23
oedipally structured couple, formation
   46
oedipal object, repressed representation
   24
oedipal organisation: fragility 47;
   observation 53, 75; sublimated
   homosexual current, direction 53;
   world of others 129
OEdipal organisation 46–47
Oedipal triangulation 18
OEdipus complex 17–18, 63; correlate
   14; couple-object, relationship 20–22;
   decline, responsibility 25; dissolution
   21; failure 21–22; infantile sexuality
   process 55; representation 17–18;
   sibling complex, link 139
OEdipus, negative OEdipus 53
offensive alliances 67; breakdown 85
omnipotence, fantasies 77
oneself, double 17

psychoanalytic process, inauguration 91
psychoanalytic thought procedure,
    basis 91–92
psychoanalytic work, ethics 12
psycho-bodily pairing, fantasy 8
psychoic bisexuality 8
psychopathological troubles 105
psychosexual organisation 23
psychosomatic economy 80
psychosomatic organisations 8
psychotic virtualities 87
pubertal blossoming 22
pubertal phases, childhood phases
    (separation) 14
pubertal waiting 14
public couple 47; private couple, rela-
    tionship 69
punishment, need 85

quasi-mutism 124
questioning process, elaboration 83–88

rapprochement 104
reality levels, functions (correspon-
    dence) 11–12
real parental couple, infantile mnesic
    representation 85
real parental objects, disinvesting 24
reassessment, capacity 114
reciprocal caring 146
reciprocal communication 121
reciprocal possession 151
reconstituted family, new couple
    (conflictual relationship) 106–107
reflexive capacities, level 114
refusal of the feminine (Freud) 52
regression: inducing 123; observation
    61; somatic regression 79
regressive movement, restructuring 13
regressive-progressive movement 75
rejection, basis 67
relational metamorphoses 43
relationships: Ego-Other relationship
    41; functioning 32; kinds, impact 36;
    psychotic virtualities 87; triangular
    relationship 37
re-libidinalisation 145
renunciation contract 66, 70
repetition 41, 56; compulsion, forms
    (diversity) 74
representation: emergence 131; function
    131; process 124
representative-affects 60
representative-representations 60

repressed contents, result 71
repression: attraction 76; impact 71
reproaches: impact 97; violence 103
resistance alliances, establishment 125
resolution modality 67
restorative investments 48
reticence, expression 98–99
retiree, psychic dynamic/economy
    (implications) 78
ritual activities, evolution 69
ritualised scenarios 77
Rosenberg, Benno 35–36, 42, 75–76
rubbish spaces 67
Ruffiot, André 77

sadistic primal scene, reactivation 124
sadistic tendencies 101
sadomasochistic punitive solution 72
same sex: identification 18; parent
    image 26
satisfaction: bisexual forms 53;
    hallucination 51; opportunities 25;
    renunciation contract 66
schizo-paranoid position, regression 60
secondarised cooperation 8
secondary narcissism 60
secondary process 62; primary process,
    imbalance 79
secondary single person, status 152
secondary structuring alliances 66–67, 70
second organising phase 22
seduction: fantasy (fantasies) 63, 130;
    masochistic seduction 113; role 82
self-eroticism 60
self-esteem, regulation 19
self, losses (experiences) 51
self-preservation 47; preservation 32
self-preserving-Eros 76
separation: forces, work 81; inherent
    suffering 86–87; oral anxiety 63;
    reflection 83–88; work 87–88, 107–108
sessions, end (determination) 146–147
sexes, difference 96
sex life, problems 99
sexologist, recommendation 142
sexual-bodily functions 11–12
sexual-bodily reality 8
sexual drives, concern 20
sexual experiences, disappointment 100
sexual genital activity, possibility 19
sexual identity 47, 49–50
sexualisation process 56
sexualised body, new image (integra-
    tion) 19

For Product Safety Concerns and Information please contact our EU
representative GPSR@taylorandfrancis.com
Taylor & Francis Verlag GmbH, Kaufingerstraße 24, 80331 München, Germany

www.ingramcontent.com/pod-product-compliance
Lightning Source LLC
Chambersburg PA
CBHW050608280326
41932CB00016B/2958